KEEP MOVING!

KEEP MOVING!

FITNESS THROUGH AEROBICS AND STEP

FOURTH EDITION

ESTHER PRYOR

MINDA GOODMAN KRAINES

MAYFIELD PUBLISHING COMPANY

MOUNTAIN VIEW, CALIFORNIA

LONDON · TORONTO

Library of Congress Cataloging-in-Publication Data

Pryor, Esther.
    Keep moving! : fitness through aerobics and step/Esther Pryor,
Minda Goodman Kraines.—4th ed.
      p. cm.
    Includes bibliographical references and index.
    ISBN 0–7674–1200–1
    1. Aerobic dancing.   I. Kraines, Minda Goodman. II. Title.
    RA781.15.K36   1999
    613.7′15—dc21
                                      99–29763
                                        CIP

Manufactured in the United States of America
10   9   8   7   6   5   4   3   2   1

Mayfield Publishing Company
1280 Villa Street
Mountain View, California 94041

Sponsoring editor, Michele Sordi; production, Michael Bass & Associates; manuscript editor, Chris Thillen; art director and cover designer, Jeanne M. Schreiber; text designer, Jean Mailander; illustrator, Natalie Hill; manufacturing manager, Randy Hurst. The text was set in 10/12 Sabon by ColorType and printed on 45# Highland Plus by R. R. Donnelley & Sons.

Cover photo: © Copyright 1998 Tony Stone Images/Lori Adamski Peek; pages xiv (top), 40, 76, 100, 138 © Karen T. Borchers; pages xiv (bottom), 10, 26 (top), 54, 114, 158 James Claffey; page 26 (bottom), courtesy Alan Rosenberg; page 64, Richard Hutchings/Photo Edit.

CONTENTS

PREFACE

We have been extremely gratified by the success of *Keep Moving!* Since its initial publication in 1987, more than 50,000 college students have found it an invaluable resource for getting the most out of their aerobic classes.

Expansive developments in the fitness and aerobics industry have dictated numerous changes in the fourth edition of *Keep Moving!* However, in this new edition, our goals still remain the same: to provide lucid, accurate coverage of the basic scientific and physiological principles that underlie aerobic fitness; to describe the most universal fitness movements clearly and with an abundance of illustrations; and to offer brief discussions of such vital topics as posture, flexibility, injuries, nutrition and stress, so that the class time can be spent moving!

The fourth edition of *Keep Moving!* expands on previous information and includes new topics to excite both the novice and seasoned aerobic student. New features include

- A new chapter that is solely devoted to step aerobics. Chapter 9 includes valuable step techniques as well as universal step movements with detailed movement illustrations.

- Revised, as well as new, student worksheets that the instructor can assign for home study. The revised worksheets are easier to follow. New worksheets expand on concepts discussed in the text.

- An expanded chapter on variations of aerobic workouts. Chapter 12 covers new exciting topics including aerobic kickboxing, indoor group cycling, and water fitness classes.
- A new website appendix features an up-to-date list of annotated website links.

Minda Goodman Kraines thanks her husband, Guy, and her daughters, Denaya and Marissa, for their love and support. Esther Pryor thanks John Silva for his continued support, understanding, and encouragement throughout the years.

We are grateful to James Claffey for his photography. We sincerely appreciate his time, energy, and talent.

We would like to express our appreciation to those who served as models for the new illustrations in this book:

Tanin Abdullah

June Brown

Stephanie Byrd

Eberechi Chindah

Julie DeBernardi

Teri Geiger

Jennifer Gobell

Dora Gomez

Lawrence A. Herzig

Daniel Marks

Peggy Gravendaal-Marquez

Andres Marquez III

Mary Napoitano

Peter Napoitano

John Silva

David Sumner

Robyn Vogel

Yumiko Wilson

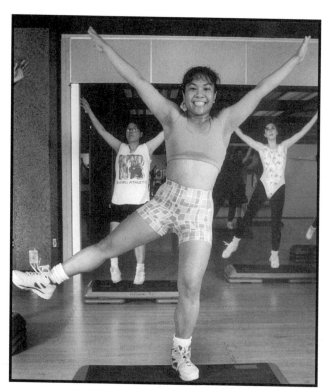

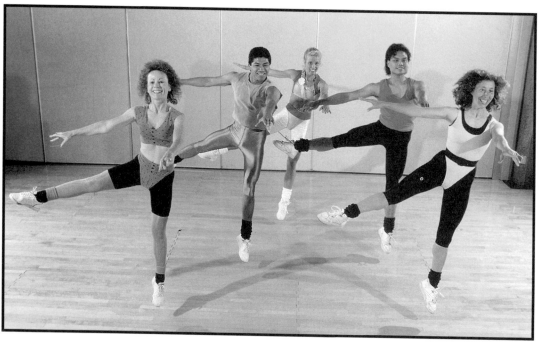

1

GETTING STARTED ON A HEALTHY LIFESTYLE

t is one thing to understand the importance of exercise and diet as a means to a healthy lifestyle, it is another thing to actually pursue and live these values. In this book, we introduce a way that can lead to a healthy lifestyle through the attainment of a physically fit body. The fit person not only exercises but also leads a lifestyle that is balanced with good nutritional habits, a well-adjusted attitude, and the ability to relax. Leading a healthy lifestyle can not only effectively prevent or delay chronic diseases but also enhance the quality of life and make a person's life more manageable.

Keep Moving! focuses on physical activity as a means to attain this healthy lifestyle. As John F. Kennedy said, "Physical fitness is not only one of the most important keys to a healthy body, it is also the basis of dynamic and cre-

ative activity." The aerobics workout is essential in helping you to achieve a healthy body. It is a successful combination of exercise and *fun!* If this is your first aerobics class, you need to know what to expect from the class and what is expected of you in the class. This opening chapter of the text describes all the details to get you started on the right path to fitness and a healthy life!

MEDICAL CONSIDERATIONS

Before embarking on an aerobics program, you may want to consider a medical evaluation of your current health status. If you have been following a regular exercise program, an aerobics class should pose no physical problem. However, certain risk factors make it appropriate for the student to consult with a physician and receive a medical clearance before embarking on an exercise program. Factors to be considered include

1. *Your age and level of activity.* Men and women over 45 who have not been involved in a regular exercise program.
2. *Pregnancy.* Women who are pregnant or who have given birth within the previous 3 months.
3. *A history of heart disease.* The severity of the condition will determine the appropriate level of exercise participation.
4. *Hypertension.* This should not deter a person from exercise, but a physician's clearance is essential.

If you are included in any of the risk groups listed above, your physician will help you decide whether you can safely participate in an aerobics class. Once you are committed to begin your exercise program, the first worksheet, found on page W-1, should be completed and returned to your instructor before you start your class. This information will provide the instructor with knowledge about your present health condition and other appropriate information to make your workout safe and effective.

STRUCTURE OF AN AEROBIC WORKOUT

Warm-Up

A warm-up is like tuning a fine instrument. The body must be tuned in preparation to responding to the demands placed on it in an aerobic workout.

Most fitness professionals highly recommend a warm-up, although there is little scientific evidence that it helps performance or prevents injury. However, the warm-up is stressed for several reasons. First, it is believed that warm-up shortens the cardiovascular and muscular systems' adjustment period to the oncoming stress of physical activity. The warm-up thus lets the body gradually shift from a resting state to an active state without undue shock.

Second, the warm-up is thought to minimize the risk of inadequate blood flow to the heart during the first few seconds of heavy exercise because it gives the heart time to adjust from being at rest to undergoing sudden, strenuous activity (14). This also helps to prevent **arrhythmia** (abnormal heartbeats) because the heart has time to adjust to the greater amount of blood supply.

The third major goal of the warm-up is to raise the body's core temperature by as much as 2 degrees. This can affect the body in many ways:

1. Increase the metabolic rate, which in turn increases the rate at which energy is used
2. Increase the flow of blood to the muscles
3. Increase the release of oxygen to the muscles
4. Increase the speed and force of muscle contraction
5. Increase muscle elasticity

Finally, the warm-up is also thought to be of important psychological benefit because it mentally prepares a person for the strenuous demands of the upcoming workout. Many experts believe that exercise prior to a strenuous activity gradually prepares a person to go all out without fear of injury. In competitive athletics, many participants consider the warm-up an activity that prepares them mentally for their event, an opportunity for them to clearly focus their concentration or to psyche up for the upcoming performance (22).

We believe that a warm-up is valuable before engaging in a vigorous aerobic workout. To attain a thorough warm-up, you should adhere to certain concepts. The warm-up is *not* a time for intense stretching; it is a time to loosen and ready the muscles for the aerobic movements to follow.

The time necessary for warm-up varies with each individual, depending on fitness level and age. Generally, a minimum warm-up of 5 to 10 minutes is adequate. Pre-warm-up exercises can help those who want more warm-up activity. For such individual pre-warm-up, allow yourself approximately 10 minutes before class.

Be sure to pay extra attention to warming up any area of your body that is weak or prone to injury.

The warm-up itself consists of three phases, which may be conducted in any order depending upon the preference of the instructor.

1. Isolations
2. Active warm-up
3. Static stretch

Isolations   The isolation warm-up phase is very short and involves simple moves (isolations) that focus on one body part at a time. This part also concentrates on posture and body alignment. The entire phase may take no more than 1 or 2 minutes, yet it is important because it helps to create body awareness.

Active Warm-Up   The active warm-up elevates your heart rate and warms the muscles. This phase starts slowly and the pace and intensity are gradually increased until your body begins to feel loose and warm. The active warm-up phase in floor aerobics involves simple calisthenics, full-body movements, and possibly light jogging or walking. In step aerobics, the active warm-up will include floor movements as well as basic stepping. Light perspiration may be an indicator that your body is ready for more intense activity.

Static Stretch   The last warm-up phase is the static stretch. A static stretch is when you take a stretch position with a specific body part to the point of slight discomfort and you hold this position for 10 to 30 seconds. Exercise stretches should be static rather than ballistic (bouncing). A slow static stretch tends to counteract a mus-cle's stretch reflex, whereas the sudden stretch of a ballistic exercise contracts the muscle, which negates the purpose of the stretch (16). Static stretching also requires less expenditure of energy, which probably causes less muscle soreness and yields more relief from muscular distress (11).

The static stretch phase consists of simple stretches of specific muscle groups that are used in aerobics. The muscle groups include the quadriceps (front of the thigh), the hamstrings (back of the thigh), the gastrocnemius and soleus (the calf and Achilles tendon or back of the lower leg), the tibialis anterior (the shin or front of the lower leg), and the gluteus maximus (buttocks muscle).

Aerobic Warm-Up

Following the warm-up, the first aerobic part of the workout, the aerobic warm-up, begins with low- to moderate-intensity movements. In floor aerobics, these initial movements, combined into simple routines, incorporate full-body movements that emphasize the use of the large muscle groups. Many of the steps will be low impact, which means one foot is always on the ground and there is minimal jumping, hopping, and jogging. Variations on walking, sliding, and lunging may be incorporated into routines that move around the room in order to increase the heart rate. In the step workout, the aerobic warm-up includes the use of low-level arm movements with basic step patterns. As the warm-up continues, basic step patterns evolve into traveling step patterns with moderate arm movements. During this phase of the aerobic workout, the heart rate and oxygen consumption will gradually increase so that, by the end of this phase, which is usually about 5 to 10 minutes in length, the target heart rate or exercise heart rate zone is achieved.

Peak Aerobics

During the peak aerobic phase, the floor aerobic workout will advance to high-impact routines and/or more stenuous low-impact moves. The step workout will utilize movements that include large leg lifts, power movements, and high-level arm patterns. All routines are designed to keep the heart rate within the target heart rate zone and can be modified to suit the individual's fitness level. The main emphasis is to "keep moving." The entire phase lasts between 20 and 30 minutes depending upon the time length of the scheduled class.

Aerobic Cool-Down

The aerobic cool-down follows the peak aerobic phase of a lesson and is designed to slowly decrease the aerobic movements to a lower intensity and slower pace. During the aerobic exercise phases of the workout, the heart pumps a large amount of blood to the working muscles to supply them with the oxygen needed for movement. As long as exercise continues, the muscles squeeze the veins, forcing the blood back to the heart. If exercise stops abruptly, the blood is left in the area of the working muscle. Aerobic movements may cause blood to pool in the lower extremities. Because the heart has less blood to pump, blood pressure may drop, which may cause light-headedness or dizziness. However, a gradual tapering off of activity helps the muscles send the extra blood in the extremities back to the heart and brain. In addition, cool-down exercises help to prevent muscle soreness and promote faster removal of metabolic waste (5, 32).

The aerobic cool-down phase should be a minimum of 5 minutes to allow the body time to recover from the stress of the peak aerobic workout. Although the amount of time needed varies with each individual, the heart rate should return to 120 beats per minute or below, and sweating should be reduced by the end of the aerobic cool-down phase (22). The transition from the peak aerobic workout to the aerobic cool-down phase is accomplished by gradually diminishing the intensity of the movements. Fundamentally, movements should rhythmically flex and extend the legs with small, simple motions. Arm movements should be kept below heart

level. Stretches specifically for the quadriceps, hamstrings, lower leg muscles, and Achilles tendon may also be performed at the end of this cool-down phase.

Body Toning and Conditioning

Body toning and conditioning exercises may follow either the warm-up or the aerobic cool-down phase of the class. This section can last anywhere from 5 to 20 minutes depending on the instructor's format and emphasis. This phase of the class does not involve cardiovascular endurance but focuses on individual muscle groups and promotes muscular strength and endurance. Exercises specifically for the abdominal region, the arms, chest, buttocks, and thighs are executed, with particular attention to body alignment and exercise technique. Resistance equipment may be used to increase the difficulty of the exercises. As with the aerobic workout, this phase of the class is also choreographed with smooth transitions between the specific exercises.

Flexibility Cool-Down

Just as the warm-up prepares the body for activity, the flexibility cool-down prepares the body for rest. This phase, lasting from 5 to 10 minutes, involves slow, sustained stretching for all the major muscles used during the aerobic workout. Deep stretching at this time is most beneficial, because the muscles are warm and can allow for the maximum stretch. Stretching at this time helps to maintain and increase flexibility and helps to prevent muscle soreness. Much of this phase is executed on the floor. A mat may be used as cushioning for the body.

Relaxation

Being able to relax is as important to the body as being able to successfully withstand imposed physical demands. Not all exercise classes include a relaxation phase, but it is certainly a welcome activity after a strenuous workout. Relaxation exercises may incorporate breathing techniques and active or passive relaxation activities. A properly designed aerobics class is a way to reduce levels of stress and a way to promote relaxation. However, the class must be within your capacity so that you are not overstressed or overworked. Your participation must not lead to chronic fatigue or cause you to become obsessive about exercise, yet it should be motivating so as not to lead to boredom or exercise burnout.

The next sections will help you understand how to work safely and effectively in your aerobics class, thus achieving the maximum benefits with the minimum stress!

REGULAR ATTENDANCE

To achieve fitness benefits from an aerobics program, you must attend class (or participate in aerobic activity) at least three times a week for a minimum of 20 minutes. These classes should be evenly distributed throughout the week, with a maximum of 2 days' rest between classes. If you must miss a class, substitute a jog, quick walk, or another aerobic activity within the week.

If you are ill or unable to exercise over a certain length of time, it is important to gradually work back to your former level of activity. It may take you three or more classes after an illness to perform with the same energy you expended prior to your absence. With regular participation, you can maintain and improve fitness levels.

INDIVIDUAL PACE

We have all heard the fitness axioms "train, don't strain" and "no pain, no gain." Somewhere between these two ideas is a middle ground that provides the safest and most productive workout pace. You are not competing with anyone but yourself in aerobics class, so it is important

to work at your level; set the pace that is most beneficial for your body. Keep breathing easily, and never hold your breath. If you can converse easily when performing aerobics, you are working at the correct pace.

In aerobics, the heartbeat is regularly monitored to help establish a pace that will produce improved fitness levels. Monitoring the heart rate also helps to prevent overexertion. Aerobic routines are choreographed so that, depending on the individual fitness level, sections of routines allow students to participate at their own desired impact or intensity level.

WHAT TO WEAR

Comfortable clothing that allows ease of movement is the appropriate attire for aerobics. The fashion industry has provided an assortment of specialty aerobics apparel to fulfill these needs. This attire includes leotards, crop tops, leggings, and bike shorts. Simple jogging shorts and a T-shirt are also acceptable for the aerobics class. Some additional clothing, such as sweat shirts and pants, can be worn for the beginning of class to provide warmth to the body until your body temperature increases. These overgarments, which superficially heat the body, should be worn only for warm-up. A popular notion is that use of these items during a workout can lead to quick weight loss, but in truth you are only sweating off water—not fat! In warm weather you should wear the minimum amount of clothing so that you can sweat freely and let your cooling system work. Because the body needs to sweat freely, cotton is the best material for exercise wear because it absorbs perspiration. As cotton becomes damp, the air evaporates the moisture and cools your body.

Support undergarments are extremely important in aerobic exercise. Women should wear a sports bra that fits snugly and provides adequate support during the vigorous running and jumping movements in class. Specific exercise or sports bras can be purchased in fitness apparel stores and in many retail clothing stores. Men should wear athletic supporters or dance belts for adequate support during exercise activities. Your instructor will usually provide guidance on aerobics attire, but if the outfit provides freedom to move, it is probably appropriate.

SHOES

Shoes are the most important investment you can make for your aerobics class. Because of the wide variety of aerobics shoes available, there are many considerations in purchasing your aerobics footwear. The following sections discuss important factors for selecting the shoe that is most appropriate for your foot.

Foot Facts

Your foot is a complicated structure made up of 26 bones, 33 joints, and about 20 muscles that control movement. There are three basic foot types; your type of foot dictates the type of shoe you should wear for an aerobic dance class.

The ball of the *normal foot* rests on the ground regardless of whether the heel is lifted. The normal foot will fit most shoes as long as the heel fits snugly and the shoe accommodates the width of the foot.

The *cavos foot* has a high arch and tends to absorb shock poorly. This type of foot needs a shoe with a firm counter (the stiff piece around the heel, usually of leather). Additionally, heel lifts may sometimes be necessary for the high-arch foot.

The *flatfoot* has a poor arch and has no rise to the top portion of the foot when viewed from the side. The flatfoot requires a very firm counter and a very firm midsole.

Shoe-Buying Tips

Shoes are the major monetary investment for an aerobics class and the most important item you wear to class. Most aerobics shoes today provide

stability at the rear of the foot, where shock absorbency and stability are needed during exercise. As you look at the many models available, keep in mind your specific foot type and consider the following points as you compare shoes:

1. Leather is the best material for aerobics shoes because it breathes and molds to your foot. A hard leather gives better support than a soft leather, which stretches after a few wearings.

2. Lateral support straps (straps that cross the upper) provide foot stability. Straps that are close to the front of the shoe (closer to the toe) provide greater support.

3. The sole width should match the heel width. If the sole is too narrow, it will not provide enough stability for your foot during landing.

4. There should be an adequate longitudinal arch support.

5. The sole should be flexible at the ball of the foot with a flexible upper also available.

6. The toe box should be high enough so you can wiggle all your toes within the shoe.

7. There should be a padded heel collar.

In-Store Shoe Test

Keep in mind the type of flooring on which you will be exercising, and try to test your shoe on a surface in the store that most resembles the one in the class. If you do aerobics on carpet, look for a shoe with a smooth tread, which will allow you to perform twisting and turning movements more easily. If your workout surface is hard, look for shoes with shock-absorbent midsoles.

Try a variety of movements to see how the shoe feels:

1. Roll forward on the balls of your feet. The shoe should bend at the same point where your foot bends. A lack of flexibility in the shoe may cause strain in the ball and/or arch of your foot.

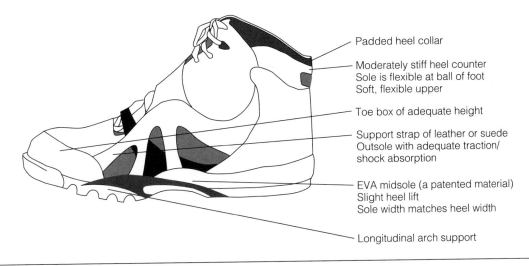

Padded heel collar

Moderately stiff heel counter
Sole is flexible at ball of foot
Soft, flexible upper

Toe box of adequate height

Support strap of leather or suede
Outsole with adequate traction/
shock absorption

EVA midsole (a patented material)
Slight heel lift
Sole width matches heel width

Longitudinal arch support

FIGURE 1-1 *Diagram of an appropriate aerobic shoe*

2. Hop on one foot to test shock absorption.

3. Stand on one foot. Keep your foot in place as you twist your upper body and hop left and right. This will cause your supporting foot to roll inward and outward, testing shoe stability. You should feel balanced as you twist if the shoe is stable.

4. Stand on one foot and raise your heel so that you are on the ball of your foot. As in test 3, twist to test shoe stability.

5. Run in place and in various movement patterns. The shoe should feel snug, but you should be able to wiggle your toes (10).

As you test several pairs of shoes, select a pair that performs the best for you. For further care of your feet, remember to wear cotton socks to keep your feet dry and free of blisters. Use foot powder or foot spray if your feet perspire heavily.

Besides proper footwear for preventing injury, the composition of the dance floor is extremely important and should be investigated when you are choosing a class. Cement covered with carpet is the worst flooring because it gives the illusion of being cushioned, yet cement is the

hardest possible surface. Hardwood flooring is the best surface for aerobics.

WHAT TO BRING TO CLASS

A few additional items may be useful in your aerobic workout: floor mat, towel, sweatbands, and light weights.

Floor Mat

A mat provides padded support for your body as you do floor exercises. If mats are not available at the class, you can buy a lightweight mat at most athletic stores, in the athletic department at a major department store, or at a chain drugstore. Any mat that is easy to carry and has some padding is sufficient.

Towel

A towel is useful in class if you perspire heavily. You can also use a towel to cover your mat, which is especially advisable if the mat is plastic because the towel will help absorb the additional perspiration the plastic creates.

Sweatbands

Sweatbands around your head and wrists help to collect perspiration. Elasticized cotton sweatbands are easy to slip on and off. You can also use a bandana rolled and tied around your head as a sweatband.

Light Weights and Resistance Bands

Light weights and resistance bands are used by many instructors as a means to create resistance during body toning exercises. These bands and weights are specifically designed for conditioning exercises and can be purchased from aerobic dance and fitness suppliers.

CHECKLIST FOR A SUCCESSFUL CLASS

1. Arrive at class 10 to 15 minutes early to give yourself time for pre-warm-up exercises.

2. Do not eat a heavy meal prior to class. Fruit, yogurt, dried fruit, or nuts are recommended preclass snacks.

3. Come to class in the appropriate workout attire.

4. Clear your mind of outside interference when you enter the classroom. Be prepared to fully concentrate on the lesson.

5. Find a space to stand where you can see and hear the teacher. Allow yourself plenty of room so you can move and stretch freely.

6. Be sensitive to any injuries you might have. Pay special attention to the injured area during pre-warm-up exercises as well as class activities.

7. Work within your target heart rate zone so you can keep moving and get maximum benefits from the workout.

8. Do not compare yourself to others in the class. Listen to your body!

9. Do not be afraid to ask questions if you are unclear about a step or exercise.

10. Bring a container of water for an occasional drink to avoid dehydration.

11. Participate in the aerobic workout to improve your fitness, posture, and knowledge of your body—and to have a good time!

Now that you know what to expect, you are probably ready to jump in and get moving. As you progress through your classes, this text will educate you on the benefits of your workout and ways to establish and maintain a healthy lifestyle.

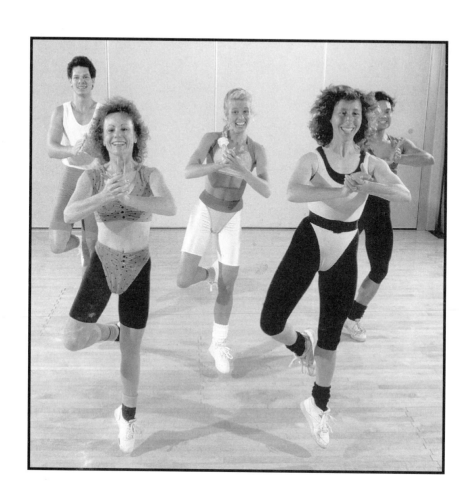

2

BENEFITS OF THE AEROBICS WORKOUT

Cardiorespiratory fitness is the most important element of physical fitness because it enables the cardiorespiratory system to carry on its functions efficiently under conditions of heavy work and physical stress. An efficient cardiorespiratory system is able to deliver large amounts of oxygen-rich blood to the working muscles over extended periods of time. The format of an aerobic workout is designed to increase the efficiency of the heart and lungs by incorporating nonstop rhythmic exercises that demand large amounts of oxygen. Thus, regular participation in an aerobic workout is one of the best ways to improve your cardiorespiratory system.

BODILY CHANGES DURING A WORKOUT

To fully appreciate the value of an aerobic conditioning program, you should understand what happens to your body during the aerobic workout and the importance and benefits of the workout. The obvious bodily changes that occur during a workout are sweating, heavier-than-normal breathing, and fatigued muscles. The internal effects from aerobic exercise are not visibly apparent; the heart, lungs, blood vessels, and the body's metabolism all undergo changes.

Heart

During an aerobic workout both the rate at which the heart beats (termed **heart rate**) and the amount of blood the heart pumps per beat (termed **stroke volume**) increase, so that the total amount of blood the heart pumps in 1 minute (termed **cardiac output**) increases. Blood pressure is also affected by aerobic exercise.

Systolic blood pressure is a measure of the rhythmic contraction of the heart as blood *leaves* the heart via the ventricles. During aerobic exercise, the systolic pressure rises with increased cardiac output. **Diastolic blood pressure** is a measure of the resting pressure in the arteries when the heart is not contracting. Diastolic blood pressure usually remains the same or slightly decreases during aerobic exercise (24, 26, 27). Blood pressure readings measure both the systolic and diastolic blood pressure. The average blood pressure is 120/80. The top number is the systolic blood pressure and the bottom number is the diastolic blood pressure.

Lungs

During aerobic exercise, the body demands more oxygen, so the lungs must deliver more oxygen to the working muscles through the blood. In turn, excess carbon dioxide must be removed from the muscles through the blood. For this accelerated exchange of oxygen and carbon dioxide between the lungs and the blood to occur, both the rate and the depth of breathing must increase (28).

Blood Vessels

During aerobic exercise, the blood vessels shift the blood flow from the visceral (abdominal) organs to the working muscles and to the skin. The muscles of the body directly involved in exercise need more oxygen and, therefore, require more blood flow. The skin receives more blood to help regulate body temperature and reduce body heat through the evaporation of sweat.

Metabolism

Metabolism is the body's process of converting food into energy through numerous chemical reactions (26). During an aerobic dance workout, as the muscles' need for oxygen increases, more energy is expended, which increases the metabolic rate (how rapidly the body uses its energy stores). Increased metabolic rate allows the body to use more energy—represented by calories—both during the workout and for approximately 1 to 2 hours after the workout.

BENEFITS OF AEROBICS

As you become regularly involved in an aerobic program, you can look forward to experiencing many of the benefits that accompany aerobic training. From the start of a new conditioning program, it will take approximately 8 to 12 weeks until changes (the training effect) will become apparent. Generally, the following changes in the body (summarized in Table 2-1) may be anticipated.

Cardiovascular Changes

With regular participation in aerobic exercise, the size of the ventricular cavity of the heart will increase slightly. This increase in the volume of the heart will in turn increase the stroke volume (the amount of blood ejected from the heart with each beat). An increase in stroke volume will increase the cardiac output—the amount of blood ejected from the heart each minute. All these changes will put less demand on the heart, because more blood will be ejected with each beat. This change decreases the resting heart rate (see Chapter 3) because the same amount of blood is ejected from the heart with

TABLE 2-1

BENEFITS FROM AEROBIC EXERCISE

Increase in heart volume	Decrease in resting heart rate
Increase in stroke volume	Decrease in rate and depth of breathing at rest
Increase in cardiac output	Decrease in body fat
Increase in capillarization	Decrease in blood pressure for the hypertensive individual
Increase in blood volume	
Increase in hemoglobin levels	
Increase in ventilatory efficiency	
Increase in muscles' ability to oxidize fat	
Increase in metabolism	
Increase in ability to exercise at a higher target heart rate	
Increase of psychological well-being	
Possible increase in lean body mass	

fewer beats, placing less demand on the heart and thus increasing cardiac efficiency. Aerobic training also enhances the capillarization of the skeletal muscles by increasing the amount of oxygen and nutrients that can reach the muscles, which also contributes to improved cardiac efficiency.

With aerobic training, the level of **hemoglobin,** a protein cell present in the blood, increases. These cells carry the oxygen through the bloodstream and into the muscles, where ATP is then resynthesized and muscle contraction occurs (see Chapter 4). Larger amounts of hemoglobin cells will facilitate the delivery of oxygen to the working muscles and make muscular contraction easier. The exercising muscles' ability to extract the oxygen from the hemoglobin and then use it for contraction will also improve with regular aerobic exercise.

A final circulatory benefit that occurs with regular aerobic exercise is an increase of blood volume. With more blood available, once again more oxygen can be supplied to the muscle cell.

Respiratory Changes

As the depth of breathing increases with aerobic exercise, the respiratory muscles involved become more conditioned. An increase in ventilation efficiency means that less air needs to be ventilated (inhaled) to consume the same amount of oxygen. Because of improved breathing efficiency, the rate and depth of breathing at rest will also improve. Once again, the trained body does not have to work as hard for the same results.

Metabolic Changes

Trained muscles oxidize relatively more fat than do untrained muscles. The mechanism responsible for this change in energy metabolism is not entirely understood, but it may involve a greater capacity of the fat-burning enzymes in trained muscles to oxidize fatty acids (29). With the body's increased ability to metabolize fat there is an increase in the carbohydrate reserve. A conservation of carbohydrates can extend your performance time and let you exercise longer and harder before you become exhausted (28).

Body Composition

Aerobic exercise helps decrease body fat because, with increased aerobic activity, the body derives energy from its fat stores. Regular participation in an aerobic training program generally reduces total body mass and fat weight; lean body weight may remain constant or increase (3).

Effect on Cardiac Risk

Although much scientific evidence supports the view that exercise improves our health and that people who exercise are less susceptible to coronary heart disease, exercise cannot conclusively be prescribed as a prevention against cardiac disease. But let's look at how exercise affects the risk factors, and then you can draw your own conclusion.

There are four primary risk factors associated with coronary heart disease:

1. Hypertension (high blood pressure)
2. High cholesterol levels
3. Cigarette smoking
4. Inactivity

Inactivity was added to the list of primary risk factors in the 1990s by the American College of Sports Medicine.

There are also secondary risk factors:

1. Heredity
2. Sex (males are more prone than women)
3. Age

4. Stress
5. Obesity

People with hypertension can benefit from an aerobics program since aerobic exercise has been shown to lower systolic blood pressure in the hypertensive individual (19). Recent research has also shown that regular aerobic exercise can lead to a decrease in total blood cholesterol levels. There are two types of cholesterol: HDLs (high density lipoproteins), which appear to be protective against coronary heart disease, and LDLs (low density lipoproteins), which appear to contribute to its onset (see Chapter 7). Exercise will increase the HDLs in the bloodstream, whereas only diet can decrease the LDLs. With an increase of HDL cholesterol, the total cholesterol ratio is lowered, and that is positive for reducing the risk of coronary heart disease (19).

As discussed above, exercise can decrease obesity by reducing total body fat. As for the other risks, exercise obviously cannot alter age, sex, heredity, or the risks of cigarette smoking. (However, cigarette smoking can negatively affect exercise by impeding the hemoglobin's ability to carry oxygen to the blood.) It's true some things cannot be changed, but exercise can certainly delay the inevitable!

Psychological Benefits

For centuries, philosophers have discoursed about the concept of the total person: an individual who has a balanced relationship between mind and body. Health professionals advocate that involvement in regular physical exercise enhances the psychological well-being of a participant by reducing tension and stress, improving sleep habits, and increasing self-esteem and feelings of vitality.

Students who have been regularly involved in an aerobics program support what health educators believe to be true. Most agree that aerobics reduces feelings of stress, and they also claim that they can handle more than one task at a time with a more positive outlook. Some people respond that they are more focused and more mentally alert. A sense of responsibility comes with regular workout participation, that is, attending classes in a regular manner, being on time, and having all workout gear, towels, and water bottles organized. In general, there is a feeling of accomplishment.

The psychological benefits of regular exercise have not been scientifically proven. Yet, people involved in a regular exercise program generally feel much better and are more positive about leading a healthy lifestyle.

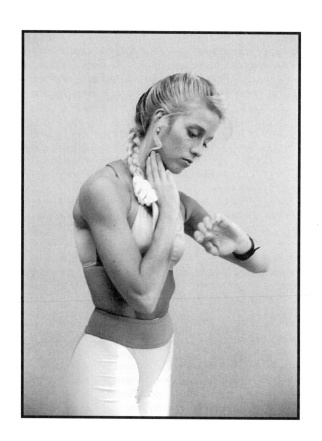

3

WHAT THE HEART
RATE TELLS US

The heart rate is the most readily obtainable measure of cardiorespiratory response to exercise. Because the heart rate is directly proportional to the intensity of exercise performed, it tells us whether we are working too hard or not hard enough. The pulse indicates the heartbeat and is counted in beats per minute. You can take your pulse at several different points on your body: the radial artery (at the base of your thumb on either arm), the carotid artery in your neck (on each side of your voice box), or at the temple in front of each ear (see Figure 3-1).

When monitoring your pulse, apply light pressure against the spot, using your first three fingers. Never use your thumb when monitoring your pulse because it has a pulse of its own and can give an inaccurate count.

When determining the exercise pulse, count each beat for 6 seconds and multiply the number by 10, or count for 10 seconds and multiply the number by 6. The negative aspect of the 6-count pulse is that a 1-count error will make a big difference in the beats per minute, whereas the negative aspect of the 10-second pulse is the difficulty in multiplying by 6. Determining the count for a short period is necessary because during a pause in exercise the pulse drops quickly. A longer pulse count, which would cause a longer interruption of movement, would produce a less accurate measure. Whatever pulse technique you use, the most important aspect is to be consistent and to begin counting as soon as possible. Some people recommend starting the count with zero as opposed to one. However, current research (1) shows that starting at zero

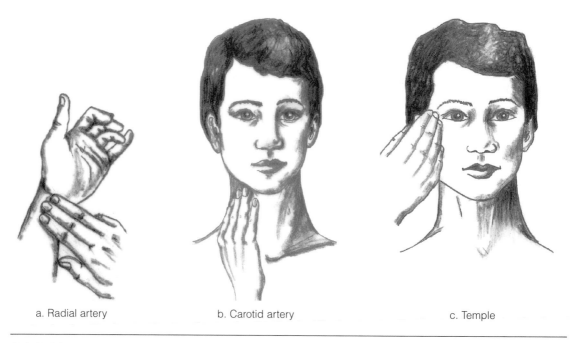

a. Radial artery   b. Carotid artery   c. Temple

FIGURE 3-1   *Sites to monitor your pulse*

is not correct if this method is the only method to be used in a group setting or the individual is not in control of the clock. Starting with a count of one is the recommended method for pulse counting in a class setting. With practice, taking your pulse during workout sessions will give you a consistently reliable measure of the intensity of your workout.

In an aerobics program, it is important to know your resting heart rate and how to calculate your maximum, target, and recovery heart rates.

RESTING HEART RATE

You should take your **resting heart rate** when you first awake in the morning. At this time, only basal metabolic demands have been made on the heart and external stimuli have no opportunity to affect the resting heart rate. In a comfortable lying position, monitor your pulse for 60 seconds or for 30 seconds and multiply the pulse rate by 2. Unlike the exercise pulse, the resting pulse rate does not drop quickly; therefore, a longer pulse-taking time will be more accurate.

Typically, after a period of 8 to 12 weeks of aerobic exercise training, the resting heart rate will be lowered (13). Medical textbooks state that the average resting heart rate is 70 beats per minute for a male and 72 beats per minute for a female. Highly trained athletes may have a resting heart rate of 40 beats per minute or lower. The slower resting heart rate means that the heart does not have to beat as often to supply the body with blood and the heart has more rest between beats. You should monitor your resting heart rate after the first 8 weeks of training to evaluate any changes. Use the chart on page W-7 to record your resting heart rate over a 16-week period.

Although regular aerobic training programs can reduce the resting heart rate, the following factors can also affect it:

Age. Resting heart rate generally increases with age.

Sex. Resting heart rate is generally higher in women.

Athletic training. Highly trained athletes usually have a lower resting heart rate.

Heredity. If there is a history of low or high resting heart rates within your family, you may inherit that trait.

Emotional stress. Intense emotional states can increase the resting heart rate.

Body temperature. When the body temperature is lower, the resting heart rate is lower. As the body temperature rises, it increases.

Smoking. Smoking even one cigarette increases the resting heart rate.

Caffeine. Caffeine intake increases the resting heart rate.

Physical illnesses. Colds, flus, and such increase the resting heart rate.

Birth control pills and other medications. These can increase the resting heart rate.

TARGET HEART RATE

When you are exercising to achieve a training effect, your heart must work hard enough to affect your aerobic capacity, but not so hard that you become fatigued. You should attempt to exercise *not* at your maximum heart rate, which is the highest heart rate you can attain and one that is impossible and even dangerous to sustain, but at your target, or exercise, heart rate.

However, you do need to know your maximum heart rate so that you can determine your target heart rate. You can predict your maximum heart rate by using the following formulas (19):

Male maximum heart rate = 220 – your age

Female maximum heart rate = 226 – your age

This predicted value varies among people of the same age group. However, the value is accurate enough for estimating your target heart rate.

Most experts agree that, for positive changes to occur in the cardiovascular system, exercise must be performed at an intensity high enough to increase the heart rate to about 60 percent of its maximum. Although no definite evidence is available, the upper limit for training intensity is thought to be about 90 percent of the maximum. For people in relatively poor condition, the training threshold may be closer to 60 percent of their maximum heart rate (29). The upper and lower limits depend a great deal on an individual's initial capacity and state of training. To calculate your target heart rate using the maximum heart rate formula, complete the worksheet on page W-8.

In 1957, M. J. Karvonen, a Finnish researcher, found from a study of young men that, for appreciable gains in cardiorespiratory fitness to occur, during exercise the heart rate must be raised by a minimum of 60 percent of the difference between the maximum heart rate and the resting heart rate (29).

Since Karvonen's findings, an increase in heart rate equal to between 60 and 90 percent of the maximum heart rate has been established as a safe and reasonable intensity. Two examples of how to calculate target heart rate with Karvonen's formula follow (see Tables 3-1 and 3-2). A complete age-adjusted chart (Table 3-3) is also included. To calculate your target heart rate using Karvonen's formula, use the worksheets on pages W-9 and W-10. You will have to determine your resting heart rate to complete these calculations.

TABLE 3-1

KARVONEN'S FORMULA FOR DETERMINING TARGET HEART RATE FOR FEMALES

Method	Example 1	Example 2
	Female 20-year-old with a resting heart rate (RHR) of 70 beats per minute	Female 40-year-old with a resting heart rate (RHR) of 75 beats per minute
STEP 1		
Estimate your maximum heart rate by subtracting your age from 226	226 −20 206 maximum heart rate	226 −40 186 maximum heart rate
STEP 2		
Subtract your resting heart rate from your maximum heart rate	206 maximum heart rate −70 RHR 136	186 maximum heart rate −75 RHR 111
STEP 3		
Multiply the answer from step 2 by 0.6 and 0.9 (60%–90%).	136 ×0.6 81.6 → 82 136 ×0.9 122.4 → 122	111 ×0.6 66.6 → 67 111 ×0.9 99.9 → 100
STEP 4		
To each figure in step 3, add your resting heart rate.	82 + 70 = 152 122 + 70 = 192	67 + 75 = 142 100 + 75 = 175
STEP 5		
The range between these two sums is your target heart rate zone to use while exercising.	Target heart rate zone = 152–192 beats per minute	Target heart rate zone = 142–175 beats per minute

It is important that you check your heart rate at various intervals during the aerobic workout. Since heart rate reflects the level of stress on the body, as long as you stay within the bounds of your target zone, you will be exercising safely. Beginners should continually check their pulse to assure that they are exercising within the lower range of their exercise zone, 60 to 70 percent. People with a year or more of aerobic experience may want to exercise at 70 to 80 percent of their training zone. More advanced aerobicizers and athletes might want to work in the 80 to 90 percent end of the target heart rate zone.

As the aerobic capacity of your cardiovascular system increases, work will become easier. You will therefore have to increase the intensity of your activities to work at the appropriate target heart rate.

TABLE 3-2

KARVONEN'S FORMULA FOR DETERMINING TARGET HEART RATE FOR MALES

Method	Example 1		Example 2	
	Male 20-year-old with a resting heart rate (RHR) of 65 beats per minute		Male 40-year-old with a resting heart rate (RHR) of 70 beats per minute	
STEP 1				
Estimate your maximum heart rate by subtracting your age from 220	220 −20 200 maximum heart rate		220 −40 180 maximum heart rate	
STEP 2				
Subtract your resting heart rate from your maximum heart rate	200 maximum heart rate −65 RHR 135		180 maximum heart rate −70 RHR 110	
STEP 3				
Multiply the answer from step 2 by 0.6 and 0.9 (60%–90%).	135 ×0.6 81	135 ×0.9 121.5 → 122	110 ×0.6 66	110 ×0.9 99
STEP 4				
To each figure in step 3, add your resting heart rate.	81 + 65 = 146 122 + 65 = 187		66 + 70 = 136 99 + 70 = 169	
STEP 5				
The range between these two sums is your target heart rate zone to use while exercising.	Target heart rate zone = 146–187 beats per minute		Target heart rate zone = 136–169 beats per minute	

OTHER TECHNIQUES FOR MEASURING INTENSITY

The pulse is not always the most accurate method for measuring intensity because of individual variability. Some people may exceed their target heart rate zone yet feel fine, while other individuals may feel unable to keep pace with the workout although their pulse is below the target heart rate zone. Because of these variations, intensity can be monitored in other ways.

The Talk Test

The talk test merely means that you are able to carry on a conversation while you are exercising. If you are breathing so heavily that you

TABLE 3-3

AGE-ADJUSTED TARGET RATE CHART FOR 60 TO 90 PERCENT OF MAXIMUM HEART RATE

Age	Maximum Heart Rate	60%	70%	80%	90%
15	205	123	144	164	185
20	200	120	140	160	180
25	195	117	137	156	176
30	190	114	133	152	171
35	185	111	130	148	167
40	180	108	126	144	162
45	175	105	123	140	158
50	170	102	119	136	153
55	165	99	116	132	149
60	160	96	112	128	144
65	155	93	109	124	140
70	150	90	105	120	135

cannot talk, then the intensity is too great. On the other hand, if you can sing a song, you are probably not working hard enough. Check your ability to talk during the class, even if it is just to count along with the instructor!

Perceived Exertion

A **perceived exertion** scale was formalized by a man named Borg in 1982. The Borg Scale (see Table 3-4) identifies the quantitative feelings of fatigue and is based on the heart rate of a 20-year-old. Subjects are asked to identify how they are feeling on a scale of 6 to 20. When using this scale, the level most appropriate for aerobic exercise is a range of 13 to 17. In Borg's terms, this is identified as "somewhat hard" to "very hard." (Beginners have a harder time perceiving their level of exertion, but as you learn the feel-

ings of your body, this scale can be as relevant a measure of intensity as the heart rate.)

Since the Borg Scale was developed, the American College of Sports Medicine (ACSM) has created a 10-point rating of perceived exertion. Using this scale, most individuals would rate themselves from 4 to 6 points if they felt they were exercising within their target range, as compared to 13 to 17 points on the Borg Scale.

RECOVERY HEART RATE

Your **recovery heart rate,** which you should take 1 minute after you stop exercising, indicates how quickly you have recovered from an exercise session. Physically fit persons generally recover more rapidly because their cardiovascu-

TABLE 3-4
BORG SCALE FOR PERCEIVED EXERTION*

Heart Rate Expected (for 20-year-old)	Perceived Exertion Rating	Description
60	6	
70	7	Very very light
80	8	
90	9	Very light
100	10	
110	11	Fairly light
120	12	
130	13	Somewhat hard
140	14	
150	15	Hard
160	16	
170	17	Very hard
180	18	
190	19	Very, very hard
200	20	

*When using this scale, the subject is asked to identify by the number listed how he or she perceives the work.

Source: Reprinted with permission from Borg, G.: Subjective effort in relation to physical performance and working capacity. In *Psychology: From Research to Practice*, edited by H. L. Pick, 333–61. New York: Plenum, 1978.

lar systems are more efficient and adapt more quickly to the imposed demands.

The recovery heart rate really has two decreasing phases: the first minute after exercise, during which the heart rate drops sharply, and the *resting plateau,* during which the heart rate gradually decreases. The resting plateau may last as much as 1 hour after exercise. Five minutes following exercise, the heart rate should not exceed 120 beats per minute. After 10 minutes, the heart rate should be below 100 beats per minute. The heart rate should return to its pre-exercise rate approximately 30 minutes after the exercise session. However, the initial sharp drop in the heart rate that occurs 1 minute after the exercise is the most meaningful indicator of fitness. To determine your rate of recovery, use the following formula:

Recovery heart rate = (exercise heart rate − recovery heart rate after 1 minute) ÷ 10

Monitor your exercise pulse immediately at the end of your workout. Exactly 1 minute after the exercise, take your pulse again. Subtract the 1-minute recovery rate from the exercise heart rate and divide this figure by 10. The higher the number for the recovery rate, the more quickly your heart has recovered from the exercise. Use Table 3-5 to evaluate your recovery rate.

The recovery heart rate also measures the intensity of the workout. Very little drop in the 1-minute pulse would indicate that you were probably working too hard and your body was having a difficult time recuperating.

Your heart rate is the best indicator for determining your proper exercise intensity. Take your pulse often throughout the workout, until you learn what your body needs to sustain your target heart rate. Remember, increase the intensity of your exercise if you are not yet in your target range; decrease the intensity if the target rate is too high. Monitor your resting heart rate periodically to evaluate the effects of your aerobic training program. Generally, a lower resting heart rate means a healthier heart.

TABLE 3-5
RECOVERY HEART RATE EVALUATIONS

Number	Condition
Less than 2	Poor
2 to 3	Fair
3 to 4	Good
4 to 6	Excellent
Above 6	Outstanding

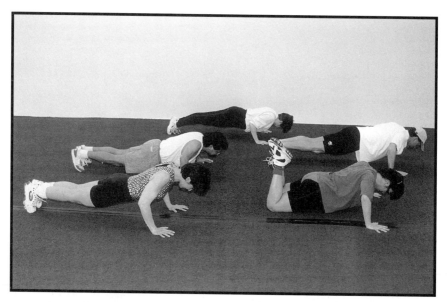

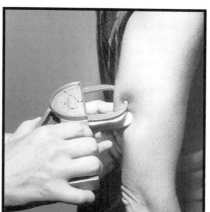

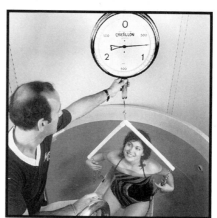

4

FITNESS COMPONENTS AND PRINCIPLES

The term *fitness* is broadly used and often vaguely defined. Many people perceive health and fitness as one and the same, yet there is a definite distinction between the two concepts. Health reflects a person's state of being; it is typically viewed as the presence or absence of disease. Fitness, on the other hand, is the ability to do physical activity or to perform physical work (23).

Health and physical education experts generally agree about the expanded (but incomplete) definition of fitness as an ability to carry out daily tasks with vigor and alertness, without undue fatigue, while still maintaining ample energy to enjoy leisure-time pursuits and to meet unforeseen emergencies.

Within the definition of fitness lie major components that are the foundation for implementing a sound fitness program. To complete the definition of fitness, we must understand the components of strength, flexibility, muscular and cardiorespiratory endurance, and body composition. It is the combination of these components that leads to the achievement of fitness. We must also understand energy production in the body and training principles.

STRENGTH

Strength is the ability of a muscle or a group of muscles to exert force. Maximal strength is when a group of muscles exerts a force against a resistance in one all-out effort (26), such as one maximum lift in a weight-lifting exercise.

The body needs muscular strength for several

reasons. First, strong muscles increase joint stability, which in turn makes the body joints less susceptible to injury (26). Second, improved muscle tone also helps prevent common postural problems. For example, stronger abdominal muscles can help alleviate postural problems associated with the lower back. Often, lower back problems occur because the strength in the spinal muscles is greater than that in the abdominal muscles; this muscular imbalance causes the postural deviation **lordosis** (swayback). Weakened muscles of the upper back can cause the postural deviations termed **kyphosis** (rounding of the upper back), and round shoulders. By building strength in the weakened muscles, these postural deviations can be modified or alleviated. Finally, the body needs muscular strength because it contributes to agility, helps control the weight of the body in motion, and helps the body maneuver quickly (26).

In developing muscular strength, the muscles must be contracted against a heavy resistance with a minimum of exercise repetitions. It is important that minimum repetitions and maximum resistance be used in order to improve muscular strength. Many repetitions with light weights will not increase muscular strength. As the muscles become stronger, the resistance applied must be increased if muscular strength is to continue to increase.

FLEXIBILITY

Although **flexibility** is generally associated with the elasticity of muscles, the total concept of flexibility is denoted by the range of motion of a certain joint and its corresponding muscle groups. Flexibility is influenced by the structure of the joint's bones and ligaments, the amount of bulk that surrounds the joint, and the elasticity of the muscles whose tendons cross the joint (26).

The range of motion of the body's various joints is called *joint mobility*. Joint mobility is measured by the amount of movement that exists where two joint surfaces articulate with each other. The greater the range of motion at the joint, the more the muscles can flex and extend. This range of motion or joint mobility is specific to each joint in the body. For example, your hip joint may be extremely flexible, whereas your shoulder joint may be inflexible (33).

There are several reasons why good joint mobility and muscular elasticity should be maintained. The movement range of muscles and joints not used frequently and regularly throughout their full range of motion becomes limited. Many movement experts claim that a lack of flexibility is a cause of improper movement performance in simple motor activities such as walking and running (26). Good joint mobility and muscular elasticity can also increase resistance to muscular injury and soreness; it is the person with inflexible muscles and joints who may experience muscular soreness or who may be more easily injured during activity because of the limited range of motion (26). However, too much flexibility in certain joints—such as the weight-bearing joints of the hips, knees, or ankles—may make a person more susceptible to injury or hamper performance. Loose ligaments may allow a joint to twist abnormally, tearing the cartilage and other soft tissue. In general, it is advisable to achieve and maintain a "normal" amount of flexibility throughout the body. Normal range varies with each individual.

For flexibility to be increased, the muscles must be stretched beyond their normal range of motion for at least 10 to 30 seconds (9). As flexibility increases, the range of the stretch must also be increased for continued improvement in flexibility. Proper stretching techniques are discussed in depth in Chapter 11.

ENDURANCE

Endurance is the ability of a muscle or group of muscles to perform work (repeated muscular contractions) for a long time. With endurance, a muscle is able to resist fatigue when a movement is repeated over and over or when a muscle is held in a static contraction (the muscle generates a motionless force for an extended time) (16).

There are two types of endurance: muscular and cardiorespiratory. **Muscular endurance** is the ability of local skeletal muscles to work strenuously for progressively longer periods of time without fatigue, such as during the execution of 50 sit-ups. Note that muscle endurance is highly specific; it will be attained only by the specific muscles exercised (26).

Using light weights and doing many repetitions of an exercise will increase muscular endurance. This task will tone the muscle but, unlike strength building, will not create large muscle bulk. Increasing muscular endurance is often termed *body sculpting,* or *body toning.*

The other type of endurance is **cardiorespiratory endurance.** This is the aspect of fitness that involves the heart and the lungs.

Cardiorespiratory (also called cardiovascular) endurance is the ability of the cardiovascular system (heart and blood vessels) and the respiratory system (lungs and air passages) to function efficiently during sustained, vigorous activities. To function efficiently, the cardiorespiratory system must be able to increase both the amount of oxygen-rich blood it delivers to the working muscles and its ability to carry away carbon dioxide and other waste products.

To enhance cardiorespiratory endurance through exercise, the activity must fulfill certain criteria. It must be of sufficient intensity, duration, and frequency, involve large muscle groups, and be continuous, rhythmic, and repetitive. These criteria are termed frequency, intensity, duration, and mode. An easy way to remember these criteria is the acronym FITT.

Frequency

Intensity

Time, which is Duration

Type, which is Mode

Frequency refers to the number of exercise sessions per week. Frequency should be monitored to adequately stress the body and to allow enough recovery time for the body to rest and adapt to the physiological overload of the workout. Typically training programs are recommended to be a minimum of 3 days per week with 24 to 48 hours of rest between workouts. Frequency is dependent upon intensity. The lower the intensity of the exercise, the more frequent training should be. Training less than 2 days a week generally does not achieve adequate training improvement in either anaerobic or aerobic capacity. If changes in body composition (loss of fat weight or increase of muscle mass) are a goal and exercise is being used for weight control, it is recommended that the frequency of exercise be 5 to 7 days per week, which represents a considerable caloric expenditure (1).

Intensity is generally defined as workload: how difficult an activity or exercise load is. Intensity may be measured by how much stress is placed on the body's physiological systems. Exercise intensity is based upon the caloric expenditure of an activity and which energy system is activated. An effective means by which to measure intensity is to monitor heart rate. The *target zone,* discussed in Chapter 3, is a term used to describe the estimated optimal heart rate suggested to provide training benefits during exercise. The American College of Sports Medicine (ACSM) suggests that intensity be 60 to 90 percent of maximal heart rate in order to provide optimal training benefits in cardiorespiratory endurance.

Duration is basically the time length of the activity. In order to achieve training benefits, duration, as does frequency, depends upon the intensity of the activity. The lower the intensity of the exercise, the longer the duration period must be. A minimum duration in which to exercise aerobically is 20 minutes at the appropriate (target zone) intensity.

Mode defines the type of activity. To achieve training benefits in cardiorespiratory endurance, the type of exercise must meet the requirements of using large muscle groups in rhythmic, continuous (nonstop) activities. Examples include walking, running, cycling, swimming, cross-country skiing, rowing, and of course, step aerobics and aerobic exercise.

ENERGY PRODUCTION IN THE BODY

To fully understand how the body responds to exercise, we must define the energy systems that occur in the body and how the energy from these systems is utilized for movement.

Our bodies require an ongoing supply of energy. This energy comes from the breakdown of the food we eat and the chemical actions in our bodies that release energy, enabling our muscles to contract. The fuel for muscle contraction is a substance termed **ATP (adenosine triphosphate)**, the body's direct source of chemical energy. A small amount of ATP is stored in our cells for immediate bursts of energy. When energy is used immediately, there is no need for oxygen to be present in the muscle cell for ATP to be used. This reaction is called **anaerobic,** meaning "without oxygen." There are two types of anaerobic energy systems: the phosphagen system and anaerobic glycolysis.

The **phosphagen system** is named after the compound **creatine phosphate,** which exists in the muscle cell. Creatine phosphate combines with adenosine diphosphate (ADP) to create adenosine triphosphate (ATP). Since there is a limited amount of creatine phosphate available to create ATP, this energy system can contract muscles for only a very short period of time, 10 seconds or less. The phosphagen energy system supplies energy needed for all-out, very intense work such as a maximum vertical jump or a maximum weight lift. Although fatigue sets in very quickly from these intense activities, recovery is extremely fast, only 2 to 3 minutes.

When energy is required for activities that are intense but that last longer than 10 seconds, either nutrients or oxygen must be delivered in order to resynthesize ATP for continued muscular contraction. For anaerobic activities lasting up to 3 minutes, the nutrient glycocose, present in our muscle cell, or **glycogen,** the stored form of the nutrient glucose, is used to continue the resynthesis of ATP. This energy system is referred to as **anaerobic glycolysis,** *anaerobic* meaning "without oxygen" and *glycolysis* referring to the breakdown of glycogen. Like creatine phosphate, there is a limited amount of glycogen stored in our muscles. As a result, anaerobic glycolysis is used only for intense bursts of energy. Windsprints or 10 repetitions of a bench press are examples of activities using this energy system.

Unlike the phosphagen system, which has no by-product, anaerobic glycolysis produces **lactic acid.** As lactic acid builds up in the cell, the muscle will fatigue and muscular contraction will become increasingly difficult. You have probably heard the term "going for the burn." This burn occurs when oxygen cannot be delivered to the cell to adequately meet the needs of the working muscle. At this point, the anaerobic energy system has been depleted. Oxygen must now be supplied to the muscle cells in order for muscular contraction to continue.

ATP produced with oxygen is termed **aerobic** energy production. Energy produced in the aerobic system is produced by two means: *aerobic glycosis* and *fatty-acid oxidation.* The initial phases of aerobic energy production will utilize the nutrient glycogen—the same nutrient that was used in anaerobic glycolysis. When exercise continues for *up to approximately 20 minutes,* is of a low intensity, and is a sustained activity, energy will be produced by aerobic glycolysis. Oxygen will combine with glycogen to produce ATP. The by-products of this energy production will be carbon dioxide, water, and heat. Examples of activities using aerobic glycolysis are walking at a brisk pace, an aerobic workout, cycling, swimming, or one of the many aerobic activities we have previously discussed.

When an aerobic activity lasts *longer than 20 minutes,* ATP is produced by the utilization

TABLE 4-1

GENERAL CHARACTERISTICS OF THE ENERGY SYSTEMS

Characteristic	Anaerobic Systems		Aerobic Systems	
	Phosphagen	Anaerobic Glycolysis	Aerobic Glycolysis	Fatty-Acid Oxidation
Fuel	Creatine phosphate	Glycogen	Glycogen	Fatty acids Glycogen
Amount of ATP produced	Very little	Limited	Unlimited	Unlimited
End products	None	Lactic acid	Carbon dioxide, water, heat	Carbon dioxide, water, heat
Oxygen required	No	No	Yes	Yes
Duration	0–10 seconds	10 seconds–3 minutes	3–20 minutes	Longer than 20 minutes
Type of activity	Maximum all-out effort: vertical jump, maximum weight lift	High intensity, up to 3 minutes: sprints	Moderate intensity, moderate duration: aerobic workout, swimming, cycling	Low–moderate intensity, long duration: marathon

of fatty acids. Fat tissue is an excellent source of energy, and fatty acids are combined with oxygen to produce ATP. As with aerobic glycolysis, the by-products of carbon dioxide, water, and heat are released with fatty acid oxidation. Any aerobic activity—running, cycling, swimming, aerobics, step aerobics—lasting longer than 20 minutes will utilize the fatty oxidation energy system. A marathon is a good example of an activity using this energy system.

During aerobic exercise, the body will use more glycogen than fatty acid depending upon the intensity of the activity. More intense aerobic activities will use glycogen, while lower-intensity activities of a longer duration will use fatty acids for energy production. Additionally, as an individual becomes more fit, more fatty acid is used for energy production. This means that a more fit individual will use more fat for energy pro-

duction, saving the glycogen stores, thus being able to exercise for a longer period of time.

The systems used for energy production are overlapping and can work simultaneously. When an activity begins, it is first fueled by creatine phosphate, and as activity continues, energy continues to be supplied by each energy system in its turn. After 3 or 4 minutes of exercise, the body must be able to supply enough oxygen to produce the ATP needed for the demands of the activity. When this occurs, it is termed *steady state*: the point at which the body's capacity to deliver oxygen to the working muscles is equal to the body's demand for oxygen. When the balance of the oxygen need and oxygen supply is equal, the balance is called a state of *homeostasis*.

Table 4-1 gives general characteristics of the energy systems.

TRAINING PRINCIPLES

In order to affect the components of fitness we have discussed so far—strength, flexibility, muscular endurance, and cardiorespiratory endurance—we must apply certain training principles to fitness conditioning. Adhering to the following training principles will help you to achieve the many benefits from participating in an exercise program.

Training Effect

The term **training effect** refers to the physiological changes that occur in the body due to regular and proper participation in a fitness program. To build a healthy body, participation in fitness activities is essential. However, unless the exercise is performed safely and effectively, the results may be minimal. To achieve a training effect and experience the benefits of exercise (whether strength, flexibility, or endurance), the individual must apply the concepts of

1. Threshold of training
2. Overload principle
3. Progression
4. Specificity principle

Threshold of Training

In developing physical fitness, there is a "correct" amount of exercise that will produce effective conditioning results. The **threshold of training** is the minimum amount of exercise necessary to produce improvements in physical fitness.

Each component of fitness—strength, flexibility, and endurance—has its own threshold of training. For cardiorespiratory training, the threshold of training is the minimal level of the target or exercise heart rate. (Remember in Chapter 3 the discussion of the training zone heart rate, which was based on 60 to 90 percent of the age-adjusted value of your maximum heart rate.) To gain optimal benefits in cardiorespiratory training, a person should exercise within the target or exercise training zone. To improve the level of fitness, a person must "overload" above the threshold of training (9).

Overload Principle

For a person to experience a training effect, selected systems of the body must be subjected to loads greater than those to which they are accustomed. This is known as the **overload principle:** A body adapts to higher performance levels and gradually increases its capacity to do more work when subjected to increased demands. The principle can be summed up in this simple "rule": Do a little more today than you did yesterday, and do a little more tomorrow than you did today.

The overload principle affects the development of strength, flexibility, and endurance. For muscular strength to increase, muscles must work against a greater-than-normal load. For flexibility to increase, muscles must be stretched beyond their current length. For endurance to improve, the workload must be sustained for an increasingly longer period of time. For cardiorespiratory endurance to improve, there must be an increased demand on the heart and lungs to sustain aerobic activity.

For the cardiorespiratory system to attain a training effect, overload must be applied to the intensity, duration, or frequency of the training program. The overload principle may be applied to a training program in five ways:

1. Increase the number of repetitions or distance of the exercise.
2. Increase the duration or time of the exercise.
3. Increase the speed of the exercise.
4. Increase the intensity or resistance of the exercise.
5. Decrease the rest intervals between exercise.

A minimum of 8 to 12 weeks is necessary for a training effect to result. Thus, even if the intensity, duration, and frequency are sufficient, most likely there will be no cardiorespiratory changes unless there has been participation in a continuous program for a minimum of 8 weeks.

Progression

Progression goes hand in hand with overload. When overload is applied to the workout, it must be done progressively, or a little bit at a time. When overloading the duration of an aerobic workout, the principle of progression would add 3 to 5 minutes onto the workout once the initial workout had reached a comfortable state. Applying progression to intensity and frequency works the same way; once the exercise has achieved a comfortable state, slightly increase the intensity or add another day to the workout regime. Never go from 2 days to 5 days all at once, or from 20 minutes to 40 minutes in one workout. Although the progression principle may appear to be a rule of logic and common sense, it is sometimes overlooked. Failure to adhere to a sound principle of progression may result in unnecessary soreness and/or injury.

Specificity Principle

The **specificity principle** (Specific Adaptations to Imposed Demands—SAID—principle) is a unifying concept that applies to all areas of fitness. It means that the human body adapts specifically to the demands placed on it. For example, strength training induces specific strength adaptations, but strength training does *not* develop cardiorespiratory fitness. Only training involving aerobic exercises produces specific endurance training adaptations (29).

The specificity principle also applies to each body part. If the legs are exercised, fitness is built in the legs. If the arms are exercised, fitness is built in the arms. For example, male gymnasts involved only in apparatus events may have good upper body development but poor leg develop-

ment (9). Finally, the specificity principle applies to certain activities—specificity of training. Specific exercise elicits specific adaptations, creating specific training effects (26). Training is most effective when it closely resembles the activity for which a person is training (9), using the specific muscles involved in the desired performance (29). For example, for an individual to improve the performance of the shot put, the person must perform both an exercise that overloads the arm muscles and a training motion that closely resembles the motion of the shot put (9). Whatever you are trying to achieve, you must train your body specifically for that outcome.

BODY COMPOSITION

A final component in determining fitness is **body composition.** All too often we judge ourselves on how we look rather than on an accurate assessment of our body's fat and lean weight composition. However, looks can be deceiving!

Body composition is generally assessed by somatotyping and by determining body fat. The body can be changed in body fat content through aerobic exercise, toning, and diet. Unfortunately, we cannot change our body type, no matter how hard we try. You can rid yourself of any obsession to look thin by understanding the body composition principles. You can also stop using the scale to determine how fat you are. Leanness is what counts, *not* lightness.

Somatotyping

People are often visually appraised as small or large or thin or fat. This description of body type by visual inspection is termed **somatotyping.** Somatotyping is the physical classification of the body. It determines the shape of your body and is something that cannot be changed, no matter how much you exercise or diet. Generally, there are three descriptive body types: endomorph, mesomorph, and ectomorph (18).

Endomorph   The *endomorph* body type is characterized by a roundness and softness of the body, with small body contours and minimal definition of muscle tone. This is generally considered the "fatness" component of the body.

Mesomorph   The *mesomorph* body type is characterized by prominent musculature and a square body shape. The bones are large and covered with thick musculature. This is generally considered the "muscular" component of the body.

Ectomorph   The *ectomorph* body type is characterized predominantly by a linear body, which may look delicate or fragile. Bones are small, and the muscles are thin, not bulging. The arms and legs are relatively long compared to the trunk of the body. This is generally considered the "thinness" component of the body.

Although body types are generally characterized into these three types, a single pure type does not really exist. Each of us is made up in part of all these three components, with different percentages of each. The dominant type that prevails is usually how we visualize our bodies.

The shape of our body still does not give us the final answer as to the fitness of our body. Nor can we rely on standard height-weight tables to reveal to us our body's fitness level. In order to complete our understanding of the difference between the weight as it appears on the scale and the way the body looks, we must understand body fat determination, which measures the body's relative proportions of fat weight and lean body weight.

Fat Weight

There are two forms of body fat: essential fat and nonessential, or storage, fat. *Essential fat* is stored in the bone marrow, in organs like the heart, lungs, liver, spleen, kidneys, intestines, and in the liquid-rich tissues of the spinal column and brain. *Storage fat* accumulates in adipose tissue, the fatty tissues that protect the various internal organs and that are found in the subcutaneous fat deposited beneath the skin. A certain amount of storage fat is necessary for maintaining health and good nutrition. Women and men need different amounts of essential storage fat.

In females, a part of essential fat includes what is termed *sex-specific* or *sex characteristic fat*. For instance, in the total mass of body fat, approximately 4 percent is attributed to breast fat tissue. The difference in body fat for females is also related to hormonal and childbearing functions. Among certain groups of female athletes with low levels of body fat, menstrual irregularities and cessation of menstruation have occurred. Generally, a healthy, adult female should have 25 percent or less body fat and a healthy, active male, 15 percent or less body fat.

Lean Body Weight

Lean body weight is the collective weight of the bones, muscles, ligaments and connective tissues, organs, and fluids. During adulthood, changes in lean body weight may occur primarily because the body's muscles are not receiving as much exercise. Although your life may be filled with activity, do not confuse that activity with exercise, which stresses the muscles. You need to regularly exercise your muscles to keep them lean and dense.

TECHNIQUES FOR WEIGHT ASSESSMENT

Simple and inexpensive methods of assessing an individual's suggested optimal body weight are the height-weight tables, Body Mass Index (BMI), and anthropometric measurements.

In 1983 the Metropolitan Life Insurance Company revised its height-weight tables, which had been used since 1953 to determine a person's under- or overweight status. The revised version of the tables included frame size determinations used to predict "ideal weight" recommendations. The Body Mass Index (BMI), calculated by taking body weight in kilograms and dividing by height in meters squared, has also been used as a tool to determine an individual's obesity level. Both of these methods are based solely upon an individual's height and weight and provide no true indication of actual leanness or fatness.

The use of anthropometric measurements provides a topographical assessment of an individual's body fat. This method uses girth and length measurements taken from various sites on the body using a tape measure. The methodology is based on the assumption that body fat is distributed at various sites of the body such as the waist, neck, and thigh, while muscle is generally located at the bicep, forearm, and calf. Height, weight, girth size, and ratios of various site comparisons are all used to calculate percent of body fat. Although better than height-weight tables or the BMI, compared to other body fat tests, this method is not as accurate.

The accurate calculation of percent body fat is a true definition of lean body fitness or obesity and so provides a sound basis for nutritional and exercise prescriptions. With the continuing interest in personal health and fitness, several methods for estimating lean body mass/body fat have been developed and are used in educational and clinical settings.

Common techniques for assessing weight are skinfold measurement, bioelectric impedance analysis, ultrasound, and hydrostatic weighing. The following sections discuss these techniques.

Skinfold Measurement

A calibrated precision instrument called a *skinfold caliper* is used to measure several predetermined sites on the body to determine the amount of body fat that lies just under the skin. The measurements we describe below—the Pollock, Schmidt, and Jackson method—are taken at three skinfold sites and provide a fat percentage based on a subject's age (see the illustrations to the right and next page) (18).

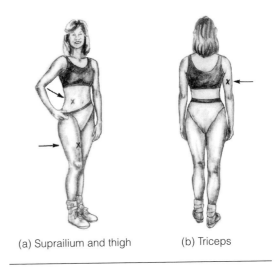

(a) Suprailium and thigh   (b) Triceps

Skinfold sites for women

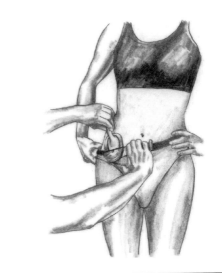

Suprailium skinfold for women: Grasp a diagonal skinfold just above the crest of the ilium, where an imaginary anterior axillary line intersects.

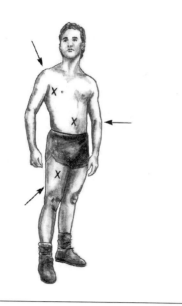

Skinfold sites for men: chest, abdomen, and thigh

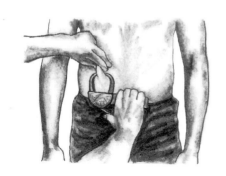

Abdominal skinfold for men: Grasp a vertical skinfold 2 to 2.5 centimeters lateral (left) of the umbilicus.

These measurements are then computed by a formula to assess the amount of total body fat. (See Tables 4-2 and 4-3.) Although this method is relatively simple as compared to hydrostatic weighing and the body composition analyzer, it

is not as accurate because it gives an estimate of only body fat, not body mass. The accuracy rate is ±5 to 10 percent of body fat. Because approximately 50 percent of total body fat lies just under the skin and the skinfold test is easy to administer, the method is widely used. It is also a useful comparative test: The original body fat measurements can be compared with new measurements taken at the same sites after months of training or exercising.

Bioelectric Impedance Analysis

In bioelectric impedance analysis, a mild electric impulse is sent throughout the body to measure body density, determining the percentages of fat and lean body mass. A computer program is used to combine the electrical measurements with the input of a person's data, including age, gender, height, and weight. Standard equations are preprogrammed into the computer software to print out an estimate of the subject's percentage of body fat.

Although this technique is easy to administer, results can be affected by dehydration or overhydration of the body, as well as by skin temperature. Predicted body fat results may be less accurate than skinfold measurement and hydrostatic weighing.

Ultrasound

An ultrasound machine sends high-frequency sound waves into the body, penetrating the skin and adipose tissue to reach the muscle. When the sound waves reach the muscle, an echo returns to the machine. The time the sound wave takes to travel back is converted by the ultrasound unit to predict a value of body fat.

Hydrostatic Weighing

Body composition can be assessed directly by a method called *hydrostatic weighing*. The hydrostatic, or underwater immersion, test is a very accurate method for determining body compo-

TABLE 4-2

ESTIMATING BODY FAT PERCENTAGES IN WOMEN: SUM OF TRICEPS, SUPRAILIUM, AND THIGH SKINFOLDS

Sum of Skinfolds (mm)	Age Groups								
	Under 22	23–27	28–32	33–37	38–42	43–47	48–52	53–57	Over 57
23–25	9.7	9.9	10.2	10.4	10.7	10.9	11.2	11.4	11.7
26–28	11.0	11.2	11.5	11.7	12.0	12.3	12.5	12.7	13.0
29–31	12.3	12.5	12.8	13.0	13.3	13.5	13.8	14.0	14.3
32–34	13.6	13.8	14.0	14.3	14.5	14.8	15.0	15.3	15.5
35–37	14.8	15.0	15.3	15.5	15.8	16.0	16.3	16.5	16.8
38–40	16.0	16.3	16.5	16.7	17.0	17.2	17.5	17.7	18.0
41–43	17.2	17.4	17.7	17.9	18.2	18.4	18.7	18.9	19.2
44–46	18.3	18.6	18.8	19.1	19.3	19.6	19.8	20.1	20.3
47–49	19.5	19.7	20.0	20.2	20.5	20.7	21.0	21.2	21.5
50–52	20.6	20.8	21.1	21.3	21.6	21.8	22.1	22.3	22.6
53–55	21.7	21.9	22.1	22.4	22.6	22.9	23.1	23.4	23.6
56–58	22.7	23.0	23.2	23.4	23.7	23.9	24.2	24.4	24.7
59–61	23.7	24.0	24.2	24.5	24.7	25.0	25.2	25.5	25.7
62–64	24.7	25.0	25.2	25.5	25.7	26.0	26.7	26.4	26.7
65–67	25.7	25.9	26.2	26.4	26.7	26.9	27.2	27.4	27.7
68–70	26.6	26.9	27.1	27.4	27.6	27.9	28.1	28.4	28.6
71–73	27.5	27.8	28.0	28.3	28.5	28.8	29.0	29.3	29.5
74–76	28.4	28.7	28.9	29.2	29.4	29.7	29.9	30.2	30.4
77–79	29.3	29.5	29.8	30.0	30.3	30.5	30.8	31.0	31.3
80–82	30.1	30.4	30.6	30.9	31.1	31.4	31.6	31.9	32.1
83–85	30.9	31.2	31.4	31.7	31.9	32.2	32.4	32.7	32.9
86–88	31.7	32.0	32.2	32.5	32.7	32.9	33.2	33.4	33.7
89–91	32.5	32.7	33.0	33.2	33.5	33.7	33.9	34.2	34.4
92–94	33.2	33.4	33.7	33.9	34.2	34.4	34.7	34.9	35.2
95–97	33.9	34.1	34.4	34.6	34.9	35.1	35.4	35.6	35.9
98–100	34.6	34.8	35.1	35.3	35.5	35.8	36.0	36.3	36.5
101–103	35.3	35.4	35.7	35.9	36.2	36.4	36.7	36.9	37.2
104–106	35.8	36.1	36.3	36.6	36.8	37.1	37.3	37.5	37.8
107–109	36.4	36.7	36.9	37.1	37.4	37.6	37.9	38.1	38.4
110–112	37.0	37.2	37.5	37.7	38.0	38.2	38.5	38.7	38.9
113–115	37.5	37.8	38.0	38.2	38.5	38.7	39.0	39.2	39.5
116–118	38.0	38.3	38.5	38.8	39.0	39.3	39.5	39.7	40.0
119–121	38.5	38.7	39.0	39.2	39.5	39.7	40.0	40.2	40.5
122–124	39.0	39.2	39.4	39.7	39.9	40.2	40.4	40.7	40.9
125–127	39.4	39.6	39.9	40.1	40.4	40.6	40.9	41.1	41.4
128–130	39.8	40.0	40.3	40.5	40.8	41.0	41.3	41.5	41.8

SOURCE: Jackson, A., and M. Pollock. Practical assessment of body composition. *The Physician and Sportsmedicine* (May 1985): 86. Reprinted with permission from McGraw-Hill, Inc.

TABLE 4-3

ESTIMATING BODY FAT PERCENTAGES IN MEN: SUM OF CHEST, ABDOMEN, AND THIGH SKINFOLDS

Sum of Skinfolds (mm)	Age Groups								
	Under 22	23–27	28–32	33–37	38–42	43–47	48–52	53–57	Over 57
8–10	1.3	1.8	2.3	2.9	3.4	3.9	4.5	5.0	5.5
11–13	2.2	2.8	3.3	3.9	4.4	4.9	5.5	6.0	6.5
14–16	3.2	3.8	4.3	4.8	5.4	5.9	6.4	7.0	7.5
17–19	4.2	4.7	5.3	5.8	6.3	6.9	7.4	8.0	8.5
20–22	5.1	5.7	6.2	6.8	7.3	7.9	8.4	8.9	9.5
23–25	6.1	6.6	7.2	7.7	8.3	8.8	9.4	9.9	10.5
26–28	7.0	7.6	8.1	8.7	9.2	9.8	10.3	10.9	11.4
29–31	8.0	8.5	9.1	9.6	10.2	10.7	11.3	11.8	12.4
32–34	8.9	9.4	10.0	10.5	11.1	11.6	12.2	12.8	13.3
35–37	9.8	10.4	10.9	11.5	12.0	12.6	13.1	13.7	14.3
38–40	10.7	11.3	11.8	12.4	12.9	13.5	14.1	14.6	15.2
41–43	11.6	12.2	12.7	13.3	13.8	14.4	15.0	15.5	16.1
44–46	12.5	13.1	13.6	14.2	14.7	15.3	15.9	16.4	17.0
47–49	13.4	13.9	14.5	15.1	15.6	16.2	16.8	17.3	17.9
50–52	14.3	14.8	15.4	15.9	16.5	17.1	17.6	18.2	18.8
53–55	15.1	15.7	16.2	16.8	17.4	17.9	18.5	19.1	19.7
56–58	16.0	16.5	17.1	17.7	18.2	18.8	19.4	20.0	20.5
59–61	16.9	17.4	17.9	18.5	19.1	19.7	20.2	20.8	21.4
62–64	17.6	18.2	18.8	19.4	19.9	20.5	21.1	21.7	22.2
65–67	18.5	19.0	19.6	20.2	20.8	21.3	21.9	22.5	23.1
68–70	19.3	19.9	20.4	21.0	21.6	22.2	22.7	23.3	23.9
71–73	20.1	20.7	21.2	21.8	22.4	23.0	23.6	24.1	24.7
74–76	20.9	21.5	22.0	22.6	23.2	23.8	24.4	25.0	25.5
77–79	21.7	22.2	22.8	23.4	24.0	24.6	25.2	25.8	26.3
80–82	22.4	23.0	23.6	24.2	24.8	25.4	25.9	26.5	27.1
83–85	23.2	23.8	24.4	25.0	25.5	26.1	26.7	27.3	27.9
86–88	24.0	24.5	25.1	25.7	26.3	26.9	27.5	28.1	28.7
89–91	24.7	25.3	25.9	26.5	27.1	27.6	28.2	28.8	29.4
92–94	25.4	26.0	26.6	27.2	27.8	28.4	29.0	29.6	30.2
95–97	26.1	26.7	27.3	27.9	28.5	29.1	29.7	30.3	30.9
98–100	26.9	27.4	28.0	28.6	29.2	29.8	30.4	31.0	31.6
101–103	27.5	28.1	28.7	29.3	29.9	30.5	31.1	31.7	32.3
104–106	28.2	28.8	29.4	30.0	30.6	31.2	31.8	32.4	33.0
107–109	28.9	29.5	30.1	30.7	31.3	31.9	32.5	33.1	33.7
110–112	29.6	30.2	30.8	31.4	32.0	32.6	33.2	33.8	34.4
113–115	30.2	30.8	31.4	32.0	32.6	33.2	33.8	34.5	35.1
116–118	30.9	31.5	32.1	32.7	33.3	33.9	34.5	35.1	35.7
119–121	31.5	32.1	32.7	33.3	33.9	34.5	35.1	35.7	36.4
122–124	32.1	32.7	33.3	33.9	34.5	35.1	35.8	36.4	37.0
125–127	32.7	33.3	33.9	34.5	35.1	35.8	36.4	37.0	37.6

SOURCE: Pollock, M. L., D. H. Schmidt, and A. S. Jackson. Measurement of cardiorespiratory fitness and body composition in the clinical setting. *Comprehensive Therapy* 6(9): 12–27, 1980. Published with permission of the Laux Company, Inc., Harvard, Mass.

sition. A person is weighed under water to determine body density: The more bone and muscle the person has, the more easily the person sinks. Because fat floats, the more fat a person has, the less the person weighs under water.

The underwater weighing technique is based on the use of Archimedes' principle, which states that an object immersed in fluid loses an amount of weight in water equivalent to the weight of the fluid that is displaced. The density can be determined indirectly by measuring the change in weight when the object (person) is fully immersed (18).

Hydrostatic weighing is not as simple as it sounds and is usually unavailable to most people because it is expensive and involves sophisticated laboratory equipment. You may inquire about this technique at colleges and universities; many schools use it in their physical fitness education programs.

SUMMARY

In your goal to achieve fitness and a healthy lifestyle you will need to address all five of the fitness components discussed in this chapter: strength, flexibility, muscular and cardiorespiratory endurance, and body composition. Additionally, as you continue in your fitness training you will want to regularly reassess your workout programs, reviewing your exercise sessions to be sure you are addressing the key criteria of FITT. There are a variety of tests that measure the five components of fitness. Use the worksheet "Fitness Profile" on page W-3 to access and record your current levels of fitness. Repeat these tests 8 to 12 weeks after the initial assessment to determine improvements.

Read on in the text to discover more about yourself and the way to fitness.

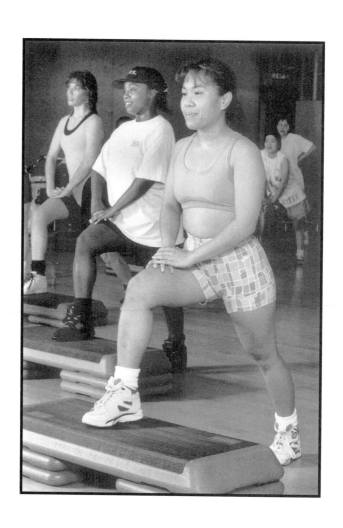

5

POSTURE PERFECT—
OR IMPERFECT?

The importance of good posture is not simply a function of aesthetics. Good posture is the basis for effective and efficient movement patterns. It helps prevent injury. It minimizes excess stress and fatigue on the postural muscles. Finally, aesthetically, it creates the best body image. Because there are so many variations in body types, there is always disagreement on what really is "ideal posture." In this chapter we will look at our body's alignment and attempt to define a body posture that is effective and efficient for all body types.

POSTURE, BODY ALIGNMENT, AND PLACEMENT

When defining **posture**, we are referring specifically to the position of the entire body in space. A person can take many different postures, yet they might not all be properly aligned. **Align-ment,** on the other hand, refers specifically to the relationship of the individual body segments to each other. We look at the alignment of the spine in relationship to the head and the legs. **Place-ment** is viewed as where the body is weighted in the space. You know from experience that, without visibly changing your position, you can shift your weight from the front of your foot to your heels. This weight shift is referred to as the placement of the body. Correct placement is critical for efficient and effective movement.

Posture, alignment, and placement are the basics of movement. Of these three, alignment is the most fundamental because it defines the position of the body before movement begins. When aligning the body, we want there to be a minimum amount of strain on the muscles and ligaments attached to the weight-bearing joints. When your body is misaligned, not only will the surrounding muscles fatigue more quickly, there is also a greater risk of injury to that body segment.

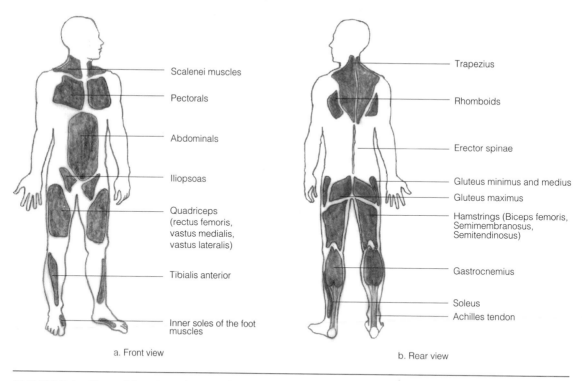

a. Front view

b. Rear view

FIGURE 5-1   *General location of postural muscles*

Correct alignment depends on a balanced relationship between the front (anterior) and the back (posterior) postural muscles. Most of the large muscles in the body are involved with the body's maintenance of correct alignment. These muscles are classified as the *anteroposterior antigravity muscles* and are identified in Figure 5-1. The antigravity musculature helps the body adequately resist the pull of gravity so it can maintain an erect posture. These muscles must be well conditioned to withstand the stresses gravity imposes and to resist the skeletal framework's tendency to collapse with the force of gravity.

The downward pressure of gravity tends to make the skeletal framework misalign at three principal areas: the ankles, knees, and hips. To counteract this effect, the anteroposterior muscles must maintain a muscular tension balance. The muscles that maintain lower limb balance are the gastrocnemius and soleus at the ankle, the rectus femoris at the knee, and the gluteus

maximus at the hip. The trunk is held erect by the erector spinae muscles running from the base of the skull to the sacrum. To balance the trunk's posterior aspect, the abdominals maintain the proper relationship between the rib cage and pelvis on the body's anterior aspect (16). An unbalanced relationship among these muscles will cause postural deviations.

ALIGNMENT REFERENCE POINTS

Basic body structure is, of course, determined by the skeleton. Figure 5-2 shows the major structural elements from the front. Figure 5-3 shows them from the back. Every individual's body structure is different, but there are visual guidelines for evaluating alignment. Figure 5-4 shows a side view of a body in correct alignment. The

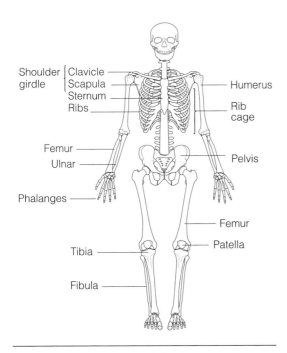

FIGURE 5-2 *Important skeletal structures, front view*

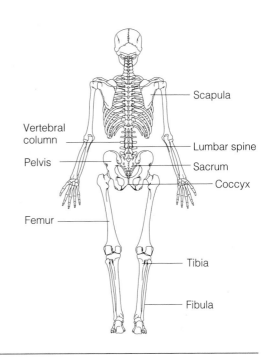

FIGURE 5-3 *Important skeletal structures, rear view*

dotted line in the figure represents the line of gravity, which pulls straight down on the body. In a correctly aligned body, the line passes through the specific points shown in the figure. These points, called *alignment reference points*, are

    The top of the ear
    The middle of the shoulder girdle
    The center of the hip
    The back of the kneecap
    The front of the anklebone

Figure 5-4 shows that the spine is naturally curved. Figure 5-5 shows the curves more clearly. The two most evident curves are in the neck and lower back. These curves absorb the shock of normal movement and protect the upper body from jarring. Do not try to eliminate or exaggerate the natural curves. The dangers of doing so range from postural deviation to serious nerve and organ damage.

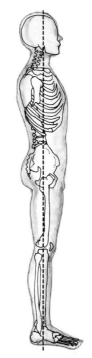

FIGURE 5-4 *Line of gravity, side view*

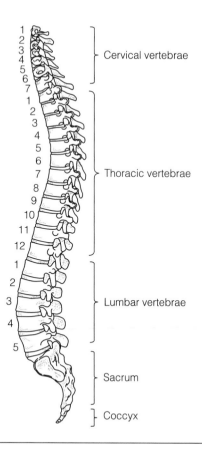

FIGURE 5-5   *The spine, with its natural curves.*
SOURCE: Adapted from Aerobic Dance—Exercise
Instructor Manual *(San Diego: Idea Foundation,
1987), 41.*

Figure 5-6 shows a correctly aligned body
from the back. The line of gravity passes through
the following alignment reference points:

The center of the head

The midpoint of all vertebrae

The cleft of the buttocks

Midway between the heels

CORRECT ALIGNMENT

Now consider the correctly aligned body in detail, from head to toe.

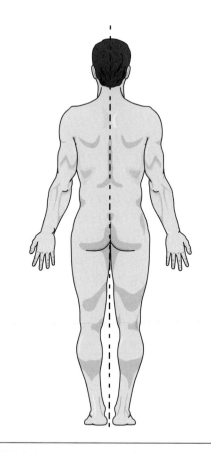

FIGURE 5-6   *Line of gravity, back view*

Head and Neck

The head, the heaviest body segment, rests on the
neck, which is a small, flexible segment. The head
should be carried directly atop the neck, not
ahead of or behind it. There should be a sense of
the neck stretching away from the spine so that
both the back and the front of the neck are long.
With the head and neck in correct alignment, a
vertical line can be drawn from the top of the ear
to the middle of the shoulder girdle.

Shoulder Girdle

The shoulder girdle—consisting of the clavicle
in front and the scapula in back—should be

directly above the rib cage. The shoulder girdle is attached to the trunk only at the sternum (breastbone), allowing it to move freely. The shoulders should not be pulled back or allowed to slump forward; they should point directly to the side so that the chest is not collapsed and the shoulder blades are not pinched. The arms should hang freely in the sockets. The shoulders should be low enough and the neck "long" enough to maximize the distance between the shoulders and the ears.

Rib Cage

The rib cage floats above the pelvis and is connected in back to the spinal column. The rib cage should be pulled in toward the spine and lifted upward from the pelvis to create a long-waisted appearance.

Pelvis and Lower Back

The pelvis is the keystone of the skeleton. The tilt of the pelvis affects the posture of the entire body and the distribution of the body's weight over the feet. To be correctly placed, the pelvis should be in a neutral position—neither tilted excessively forward nor backward—which lengthens the lumbar spine and shortens the abdominal muscles. Extreme forward or backward tilting of the pelvis can injure the lumbar spine and muscles of the lower back.

When the pelvis tilts forward, the lumbar area of the lower spine is forced to curve abnormally. The posterior discs located between the vertebrae are depressed, which results in lower back pain. When the pelvis is tilted backward, the natural lumbar curve is flattened. Anterior (forward) and posterior (backward) tilt can be rectified by proper conditioning of the vertebrae column and pelvic musculature.

Knees

The knee position, which is affected by the placement of the pelvis, should be directly above and in line with the direction of the toes. In the

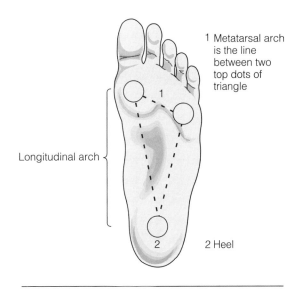

1 Metatarsal arch is the line between two top dots of triangle

Longitudinal arch

2 Heel

FIGURE 5-7 *Weight-bearing areas in the foot*

standing position, the knees should be slightly relaxed. Hyperextension (a locking or pressing too far back) of the knees is a common error.

Feet

Although the pelvis is the keystone of the skeletal structure, the feet provide the main base of support. In a static position, the greatest support is achieved when the weight of the body is equally distributed over the metatarsal arch—the base of the big toe to the base of the small toe—and the heel (see Figure 5-7). All the toes should remain in contact with the floor to provide the widest possible base of support. In addition, the longitudinal arch should be well lifted to prevent the ankle from rolling inward.

POSTURAL DEVIATIONS

When the body does not maintain correct alignment, postural deviations will occur. Since posture and body alignment are habits, most people are not even aware of their postural deviations. When you have maintained a misaligned spine

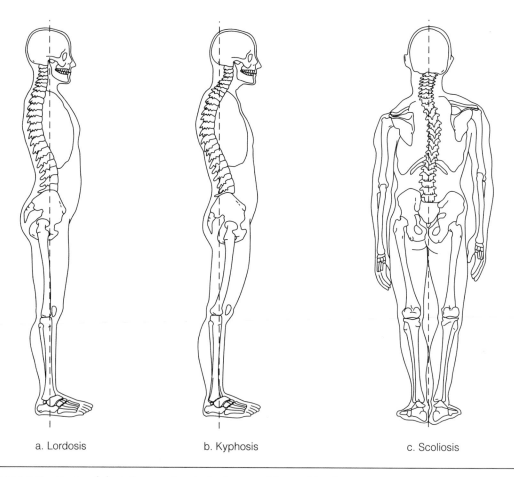

a. Lordosis   b. Kyphosis   c. Scoliosis

FIGURE 5-8   *Postural deviations. a. Lordosis: Increased inward lumbar curve from neutral; b. Kyphosis: Increased outward thoracic curve from neutral; c. Scoliosis: Lateral spinal curves with possible vertebral rotation.*

for 20 years and someone attempts to help you find correct alignment, this new position will feel odd and uncomfortable and certainly not "correct." It takes both muscle reconditioning and kinesthetic awareness of the correct placement in order to make a change in a person's posture and alignment. By giving appropriate kinesthetic cues, practicing the correct body position, and then performing specific exercises on a regular basis to stretch and strengthen the misused muscles, an individual will be able to improve their alignment.

There are three primary postural deviations. All are concerned with the alignment of the spinal column. All three can be temporary or permanent. They may be caused by fatigue or by a muscle, tendon, or ligament imbalance, all of which exercise and awareness can improve. If these deviations are caused by structural abnormalities of the bones, then exercise will not improve the condition. In this case, a physician should be consulted.

In correct alignment, there is a natural or "neutral" curve in the spinal column (see Figure

5-8). This minimizes excess stress on the spine and its surrounding soft tissues. In the deviations, the neutral curve becomes excessive. The three deviations are lordosis, kyphosis, and scoliosis (see Figure 5-8).

Lordosis is an excessive curve of the lower or lumbar spine. In this position, the pelvis has an increased anterior tilt, which increases the normal inward curve of the lower back. This spinal deviation is often accompanied by a protruding abdomen and buttocks, rounded shoulders, and a forward head. Usually poor postural habits or jobs where we stand all day can cause this excessive curve. For these situations, exercise and awareness can help greatly to improve the alignment.

Kyphosis is an increase in the normal outward curve of the thoracic vertebrae. This increased curve is often accompanied by round shoulders, a sunken chest, and a forward head. Poor habits are the main reason for this deviation. Sitting at a desk for many hours in a day can exaggerate this posture. Exercise can help to improve this problem.

Scoliosis is a lateral curve of the spine. It cannot be seen from the profile like the other two deviations. In scoliosis, the vertebrae may rotate, causing a backward shift of the rib cage to one side. The pelvis, as well as the shoulders, may appear uneven (4). Often, this deviation is structural. If this is the case, a physician should be seen to offer guidance.

If you were to carefully analyze how you stand, sit, carry and lift objects, and even sleep, you would understand how poor postural habits develop. By performing activities with a minimum of strain on our joints and muscles, we can improve our alignment and decrease our risk for lower back pain. To see change in your posture, we know that three things must take place:

1. Kinesthetic awareness of the correct alignment
2. Muscle reconditioning of the imbalanced muscles
3. Performing daily tasks with correct form

DO'S AND DON'TS FOR CORRECT POSTURE

Being aware of good alignment and maintaining good posture during your aerobics workout is very important. It is also necessary to perform daily activities in good form. Since we stand, sleep, and sit so many hours of the day, it is important to be aware of our posture at these times. We have outlined ways to improve your daily habits so that good habits result and poor posture will disappear!

Standing

- Use a footrest when standing over a step or stool; it relieves the excessive lumbar curve.
- Never bend over a table or desk without bending your knees

Lifting

- When lifting objects, always bend the knees and the hips; never bend from the waist with the legs straight.
- When holding heavy objects, always hold them close to your body; never hold them away from your body.

Sitting

- Use a special ergonomic chair, which is the best for maintaining good sitting posture, or a straight, hard chair.
- Relieve back strain by sitting forward, tightening abdominal muscles, and crossing legs at the ankles.
- If you have lordosis, use a footrest. The aim is to have the knees higher than the hips.
- When driving, you should sit close to the pedals. Sitting too far from the pedals increases the lumbar curve.
- If the chair is too high for you, this also increases the lumbar curve.

- Always bend forward from the hips when sitting. Attempt to keep the neck and back in as straight a line as possible.

Lying in Bed

A firm mattress is very important for good posture. If you use a bedboard, a softer mattress is acceptable. If you use a bedboard, it should be made of $\frac{3}{4}$-inch plywood.

- Don't lie flat on your back. This accentuates an increased lumbar curve.

- Do lie on your side with both knees bent.

- Don't use a high pillow, because it strains the neck, arms, and shoulders.

- Do use a pillow under your knees when you must lie on your back. This flattens the back and maintains good posture.

- Don't sleep facedown, because this also exaggerates the lumbar curve and strains the neck and shoulders.

- Do raise the foot of your mattress eight inches to discourage sleeping on your abdomen.

LOWER BACK PAIN

Lower back pain is one of the biggest problems that people with postural deviations experience. If you do feel pain or discomfort in the lower back, this last section will outline the major causes and then describe exercises to help alleviate the pain or make it more manageable.

Causes of Lower Back Pain

There are many factors involved in lower back pain. Prolonged sitting—an occupational hazard built into many jobs—can create unnecessary tension in the lower back by causing the lumbar vertebral muscles to become shortened and thus inflexible and by encouraging weakened abdominal muscles. When a sudden stress is then placed on the back during exercise or when performing a daily task, the tightened

muscles will strain and overstretch to accomplish the task, and injury and pain may result.

Another factor contributing to lower back problems is incorrect posture. When the muscles are continually held in an imbalanced position, the lower back muscles excessively contract in order to keep the spine vertical. This will eventually cause lower back pain.

Using faulty body mechanics, such as lifting heavy objects with the knees straight, is another way to put undue stress on the lower back. It is very important to bend the knees when lifting objects lower than the body. It is also important to keep the weight as close to the body as possible. The farther the weight is held away from the body, the more strain and possible injury can occur to the lower back.

Minimal physical activity, poor muscle tone, and excess weight, particularly in the abdomen, are other major factors that contribute to lower back pain. Regular exercise, with an emphasis on specific strength and flexibility exercises, will help alleviate these problems.

Weak abdominal muscles and inflexible muscles of the lower back are conditions that allow the pelvis to tilt forward, resulting in undue stress on lower back vertebrae. The following activities are important in helping to prevent lower back pain:

- Perform strengthening exercises for the abdominals and gluteal muscles
- Perform flexibility exercises for the lower back, hamstring, and hip flexor muscles
- Maintain good posture
- Execute good exercise technique and body mechanics

Outlined below are specific exercises to help relieve muscular lower back pain.

Lower Back Exercises

Flexibility Exercises for the Lower Back Muscles, Hamstrings, and Hip Flexors The *lower back muscles* are the muscles of the sacrum, connecting the vertebrae to the pelvis. They ex-

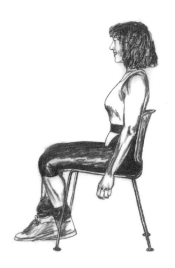
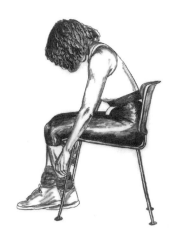
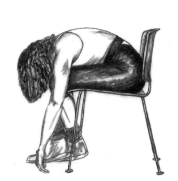

Lower back stretch

tend the lower back (arching backward) and increase the curve of the lower back. For a healthy
back, these muscles need flexibility.

LOWER BACK STRETCH

Sitting in a chair with your legs together or
on the floor with your legs crossed, exhale
and slowly bend forward one vertebra at a
time. Relax in this position with your head
as close to your knees as possible. Hold this
position for 10 seconds and then slowly
recover.

DOUBLE KNEE HOLD

Lying on your back, place your hands
under your knees to keep pressure off the
joints and bring both knees to your chest.
Stretch your lower back by pulling gently
on the upper leg, exhaling as you do this.
Hold this position for several seconds.

PELVIC TILT

Lie on your back with your knees bent,
feet flat on the floor, and hands at your
side. Slowly contract the abdominal and
buttocks muscles. The hips will lift slightly
off the floor. Hold the contraction for 10
seconds and then release. Repeat this exercise 5 times.

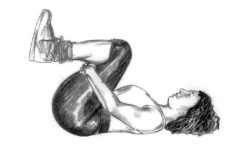

Double knee hold

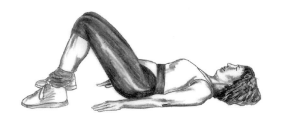

Pelvic tilt

Hip flexors are the muscles of the thighs
(quadriceps) and the deep muscles of the pelvis
(iliopsoas). They keep the pelvis in proper alignment. When they are tight, there is an extreme

forward tilt of the pelvic girdle (swayback, or lordosis). See Chapter 11 for descriptions of the quadriceps stretch and the runner lunge—a good stretch for the iliopsoas muscles.

The *hamstrings* are the muscles on the back of the thigh. They are a two-joint muscle that extends the hip and flexes the knee. When these muscles are inflexible, the curve in the lower back is increased, which causes lower back pain. It is very common for runners to have tight hamstrings. Hamstring stretches are also found in Chapter 11.

Strengthening Exercises for the Gluteals and the Abdominals   The *gluteal muscles* are located in the buttocks. They are the hip extensors. Along with the muscles on the front of the hip, these muscles maintain proper alignment of the pelvis. When they are overly stretched, the pelvis has an extreme forward tilt. Strengthening exercises for these muscles are described in Chapter 10 under exercises for the lower body.

The *abdominal muscles* also help to keep the pelvis in proper alignment. When these muscles are weak, the lower back muscles must over-

TABLE 5-1

EXERCISES TO AVOID

Region	Exercise	Modification
Lumbar and Thoracic Spine	Prone Arches	Delete, or low cobra
	Windmills	Delete
	Straight-leg sit-ups	Curl-ups
	Toe touches	Substitute sustained supported stretch on floor
	Fire hydrants	Substitute side-lying leg lifts
	Double leg lifts	Substitute curl-ups
	Flat-back bounces	Delete
	Leg lifts to rear and side above 90 degrees	Perform at 45 degrees or below
	Unsupported lateral stretch	Place hand on thigh to support back
Cervical Spine	Head drop to ceiling	Delete
	Yoga plough	Substitute gentle stretching using hand to pull head forward
	Fast head circles	Perform slowly or delete
Knee	Standing hamstring stretch	Hamstring stretch, or knee to chest
	Lotus position	Substitute butterfly stretch with soles of feet together
	Hurdler's stretch	Change knee position of bent knee to touch inside of opposite leg
	Deep lunges Grand pliés Deep squats	Limit depth of knee flexion to about 90 degrees and make sure there is no pain

compensate to keep the body erect. This causes lower back pain. Perform the abdominal exercises described in Chapter 10 to increase abdominal strength.

To totally alleviate lower back pain, the exercises recommended in this section should be performed on a daily basis. Even more important than performing the exercises is to achieve an awareness of proper body alignment. When your body knows the correct placement of the pelvis, the lower back muscles will not be overtightened but will be in balance with the muscles on the front of the pelvis. When this correct placement becomes habitual, then the lower back will be free from pain. In addition to these lower back exercises, it is also important to practice good alignment on a daily basis—and to perform daily tasks in correct form!

EXERCISES TO AVOID

To protect your alignment and have the safest and most effective workout, it is suggested that you avoid the exercises listed in Table 5-1. They are listed by region of the body most prone to misalignment and injury.

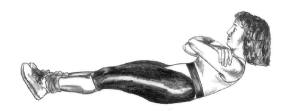

Straight-leg sit-up

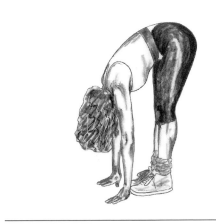

Straight-leg toe touch

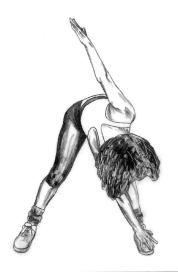

Windmill

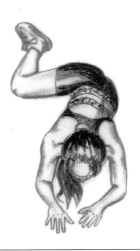

Fire hydrant

Exercises to Avoid (continued)

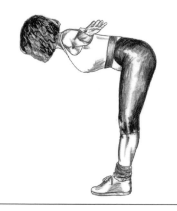

Straight-leg, flat-back bounce

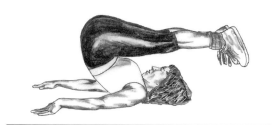

Yoga plough

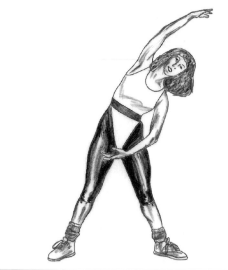

Unsupported lateral stretch

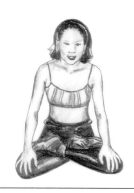

Lotus position

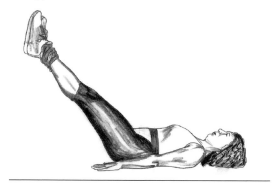

Double leg lift

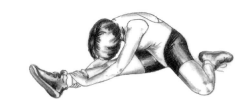

Hurdler's stretch

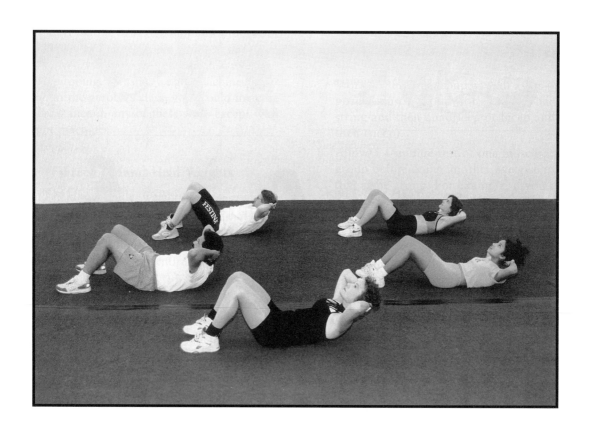

6

TAKE CARE OF YOUR BODY

Before embarking on your first aerobic workout, you should have some knowledge of injury prevention and care. You want to take full advantage of the time you spend in class. Each moment or beat should count toward improving your fitness and healthy lifestyle. Injuries can detract from a regular exercise program because they can take training time away and can affect your progress. Taking care of your body is the best way to avoid injury. Start this task by following the guidelines in the next section, "How to Survive the Aerobic workout."

HOW TO SURVIVE THE AEROBIC WORKOUT

- Always monitor your heart rate to make sure you are working at the correct intensity.

- If you have mastered taking your pulse easily, you should continue to walk while monitoring your pulse.

- Begin your aerobic workout session at low intensity; gradually increase and sustain the intensity as you reach your target heart rate.

- Make sure you are breathing evenly throughout; never hold your breath! This can cause dizziness and fainting. You should allow the breath to come in and out of both your nose and mouth at a rate that feels comfortable. The demands of the exercise will determine the rate and depth of the breath.

- You should be able to talk throughout the entire workout. If you are unable to carry on a conversation, you should lower the exercise intensity.

- Make sure you land with your knees bent on all jumps, hops, leaps, and aerial movements. Do not land with straight legs.

- Do not jog or run flat-footed. Your landing must be cushioned by rolling through the ball of the foot.

- Never come to a complete stop during the aerobic section except in the event of an injury. Slow down to a walking pace if you are out of breath.

No one cares more about your body than you do, so it is essential that you learn to listen to body signals. Involvement in any sport or recreational activity is not without risk of injury. Even when we follow the survival rules, surprises can happen. However, in aerobics, or any exercise program, risk of injury is lessened if you perform the movements and exercises with careful attention to proper technique and take certain precautions. You should recognize and follow the simple guidelines discussed in the following paragraphs. Consult Table 6-1 on page 57 for injuries that need medical attention.

SELF-ASSESSMENT

The first phase of injury prevention involves self-assessment. Evaluate your readiness to begin an aerobic exercise program. If you are not sure you have the strength or stamina, discuss your doubts with the aerobics instructor or your doctor. Ask for an exercise program that will help build your strength slowly and safely.

FOLLOW YOUR FEELINGS

Do not force yourself to exercise when you are not feeling up to it; on the other hand, do not give in to every little excuse for avoiding your exercise class. A part of all of us would rather sit and relax. Learn to evaluate when to push yourself and when to go easy.

PAIN—A FRIENDLY SIGNAL

Pain is part of your body's language; it tells you when something is wrong. When you have pain, do not ignore it—investigate it. If your discomfort is beyond normal muscle soreness and does not go away or is recurring, seek professional evaluation and diagnosis.

SORENESS

Usually the most common ailment of someone initiating a fitness program is muscle soreness. When you begin an activity to which your body is not accustomed, you can expect a slight feeling of soreness. There are two different types of soreness. *General* or *acute soreness* occurs during or immediately after an exercise session and disappears in 3 to 4 hours. Acute soreness is thought to be induced by an inadequate blood flow to the exercising muscles (*ischemia*). This condition causes lactic acid and potassium end products to accumulate; this accumulation eventually stimulates pain receptors. When there is adequate blood flow to the active muscles, these end products are diffused and soreness diminishes.

The second type of soreness is *delayed muscle soreness,* which increases for 2 to 3 days following exercise and then diminishes until it disappears completely after 7 days. The four popular theories about the etiology of delayed muscle soreness are lactic acid accumulation, muscle spasms, torn muscle tissues, and damaged connective tissues.

The degree of delayed muscle soreness is related to the type of muscular contractions. During eccentric contractions, a muscle contracts as it lengthens. During concentric contractions, a muscle shortens as it contracts. Maximum soreness seems to be related to eccentric contractions (20).

You can help prevent some soreness by

TABLE 6-1

CARE OF COMMON EXERCISE INJURIES

Injury	Symptoms	Cause	Treatment
Muscle cramp	Painful, spasmodic contraction usually felt back of leg and front of thigh.	Fatigue; muscle tightness; fluid, salt, or potassium imbalance from profuse sweating.	Gently stretch or massage area. Drink water and take potassium.
Muscle strain	Muscle tenderness and possible swelling.	Sudden contraction of muscle and poor flexibility.	Ice immediately. See physician if it does not improve.
Shinsplints	Pain on anterior aspect of lower leg. Possible swelling.	Jogging or jumping on hard surfaces, improper shoes, muscle imbalance.	RICE
Plantar fascitis	Chronic pain and inflammation to the foot, especially the heel. Longitudinal arch may also feel pain.	Overuse by putting too much stress on foot.	RICE. See physician.
Ankle sprain	Swelling, inflammation, point tenderness, swelling.	Unstable landings, rolling over on ankle.	Ice immediately. See physician.
Achilles tendinitis	Inflammation of the Achilles tendon. Pain is felt when running.	Overuse one too many times.	RICE. See physician.
Chondromalacia patella	Vague pain in knees when walking, running, or stair climbing.	Improper shoes, poor running surfaces, abrupt changes in training routine, muscle imbalances.	RICE. See physician.
Patellar tendinitis	Pain, tenderness, and inflammation below kneecap.	Repetitive jumping and landing activities.	RICE. See physician.
Stress fracture	Chronic pain and swelling. Usually occurs in the shins or ball of foot.	Repetitive jogging, jumping, and landing.	RICE. See physician.

1. Warming up properly

2. Avoiding bouncing-type (ballistic) stretching

3. Progressing slowly into your aerobic workout

4. Cooling down properly with adequate stretching

Expect some soreness if you have been inactive before starting your exercise program. Use sensible judgment regarding your body. Do not stop exercising merely because you are a little sore; the soreness will only recur later when you resume your exercise program.

SIGNS OF OVERTRAINING

We have already discussed how important it is to measure intensity and to work correctly and effectively in class. If we always followed this precaution, we would never experience signs of overtraining. There are times though when students can get carried away with the enthusiasm of the class and forget to pay attention to their heart rate or perceived exertion. Working beyond the recommended intensity level of your target training zone may cause one or more of the following *acute* or immediate signs of overtraining:

1. Rapid breathing and inability to talk
2. Profuse sweating
3. Extreme redness in the face
4. Inability to keep up with the basic class movements
5. Dizziness or light-headedness

If any of these symptoms should occur, you should immediately slow down your activity and decrease the intensity of the moves.

Lower the intensity of aerobic dance movements by

1. Decreasing the size or range of the movements
2. Lessening the use of the arms or lowering the arm movements to below heart level
3. Slowing down the movements

If you stay within your appropriate exercise range, you will maintain a positive attitude toward exercise: Workout, *don't* burn out!

There are also signs of overtraining that occur after the workout is over. These are termed *chronic* signs of overtraining. If you notice any of the following, a break from exercise or a reduction in intensity or duration might be appropriate:

1. Increase in resting heart rate
2. Chronic fatigue
3. Lack of motivation
4. Inability to relax

5. Extreme muscle soreness and stiffness the day after a workout
6. Decrease in body weight when no effort to decrease weight is being made
7. Lowered general physical resistance, such as a continuous cold or headache
8. Loss of appetite
9. Constipation or diarrhea
10. Unexplained drop in athletic performance (17)

EXERCISE CONSIDERATIONS FOR SPECIAL CONDITIONS

How and when we exercise can also be a precaution for preventing injury and pain. At certain times in our life we need to be more attentive to our body needs than other times. Think about the following situations:

With Pain from a Previous Injury

If you are recovering from an injury, you should carefully monitor the intensity of the exercise during the rehabilitation period. Although slight discomfort may be felt as you renew your exercise program, you should not feel pain per se. If pain does occur, *stop* the exercise, giving your body more time to heal. You may want to choose an alternative exercise that does not affect the injury.

With a Cold

This is a very individual situation. Sometimes, with a slight cold, exercise may help to relieve some of the aches and pains and make you feel better. A severe cold, on the other hand, could leave you without adequate strength and energy required for medical recovery. If indeed you do decide to exercise, remember to check your heart rate and exercise at a moderate workout level. Fluids are extremely important. Juices high in vitamin C are good to drink before or after the workout. If you are uncomfortable during the workout, *stop!* Resume your exercise program when you are in better health.

During Your Menstrual Cycle

As a general rule, there is no problem with exercising during menstruation. In fact, it can help to improve blood circulation which may make you feel more energetic. In some cases though, with heavy cramping, if it is very uncomfortable to move, rest is encouraged. In this case, it is advisable to see a physician to help you through the pain.

In the Heat

When you exercise in the heat, your body has a more difficult time dissipating the internal heat because the external environment does not supply any relief. Profuse sweating often results and with it, a large amount of water loss. This could result in dehydration and, more seriously, heat exhaustion or heat stroke. It is acceptable, though, to exercise in the heat; yet the following precautions must be taken:

1. Decrease the intensity of exercise beyond 30 minutes.
2. Exercise in the early morning or late evening.
3. Drink plenty of fluids before, during, and after exercising.
4. Wear lightweight and well-ventilated clothing to expose as much skin as possible to aid in the evaporation of sweat.

In the Cold

Generally, exercising in the cold poses few problems if you are prepared. Usually, in this environment the body stays cool and refreshed, but chilling can occur quickly if the body surface is wet with sweat and the dilation of the blood vessels continues to bring body heat to the skin.

Therefore, after exercise you need to retain body heat. The following guidelines will prevent problems when exercising in a cold climate:

1. Wear several layers of clothing that can be removed and replaced as needed.
2. Allow for adequate ventilation of sweat. If evaporation of sweat does not occur, the wet garments will drain the body of heat during rest periods.
3. Drink plenty of fluids, just as in the heat. Urine production increases in the cold, making fluid replacement important.

RICE: THE RECIPE FOR FIRST AID

As an athlete, you face the risk of injury. Some athletic injuries merely require self-care treatment. However, other injuries require proper first aid treatment or, depending on their severity, professional diagnosis and treatment. Apply first aid as soon as you incur an injury. Immediate treatment quickens the healing process. A simple way to remember the first aid treatment is to keep in mind the acronym RICE:

Rest

Ice

Compression

Elevation

Rest. Stop using the injured area as soon as you experience pain.

Ice. Ice reduces swelling and alleviates pain. Apply ice immediately to the injured area for 15 to 20 minutes several times a day for the first 24 hours after the injury has occurred. Let the injured body part regain its normal body temperature between icings.

Compression. Firmly wrap the injured body part with an elastic or compression bandage between icings. (A change in color or sensation in the extremities may mean the bandage is wrapped too tightly.)

Elevation. Raise the injured part above heart level to decrease the blood supply to the injured area.

You must let an injury heal completely before resuming activity. Once the injury has healed, reinitiate your aerobics training *slowly* so there will be no reinjury.

SELF-CARE INJURIES

The following injuries may require first aid treatment. If the injury does not heal with first aid treatment, consult a physician.

Stitch Pain

A pain in the side from running is called a *stitch pain,* which is the result of a spasm in the diaphragm. A stitch pain usually occurs when too much has been demanded from the diaphragm without proper preparation, that is, a proper warm-up. A stitch pain may also be due to a lack of oxygen and/or a buildup of carbon dioxide from poor rhythmical breathing. Although many instructors advise running through a stitch pain, this is *not* recommended because more muscle fibers of the diaphragm may become involved and thus increase the strain on the diaphragm.

There are two ways to get rid of a side stitch: bend over in the direction of the stitch or merely walk. If the spasm releases, gradually increase your speed from a jog to a full run. If the stitch pain persists or returns, *stop!*

Blister

A *blister,* caused by friction, is an escape of tissue fluid from beneath the skin's surface. You should not pop or drain a blister unless it interferes with your daily activity to the point where it absolutely has to be drained. If this is the case, clean the area affected with antiseptic. Then lance the blister with a sterile needle at several points and forcibly drain it. As the blister dries, leave the skin on for protection until the area of the blister forms "new" skin; then clip away the dead skin. You can prevent most blisters by taking sensible care of your feet and wearing properly fitting footwear (see Chapter 1 for tips on buying aerobic shoes).

Cramp

A *cramp* is a painful spasmodic muscle contraction. Muscle cramps commonly occur in the back of the lower leg (calf), the back of the upper leg (hamstring muscle group), and the front of the upper leg (quadriceps muscle group). Cramps are related to fatigue; muscle tightness; or fluid, salt, and potassium imbalance (12). To relieve the pain, gently stretch or massage the cramped muscle area. Since muscle cramps can be caused by a fluid and mineral imbalance from profuse sweating, drink water freely and increase your potassium intake naturally with foods such as tomatoes, bananas, and orange juice.

Muscle Strain

One type of muscle strain is the muscle pull, or damage to the muscle tissue. Scar tissue forms in the damaged area, and—because scar tissue is not as resilient as muscle tissue—you feel the effect of the pull for a long time. Another type of muscle strain involves the tissue around the muscle. For example, the tendons—the tissues that attach muscles to bones—often sustain strains. The blood supply to muscle-surrounding tissues is smaller than to the muscles; therefore, strains in these tissues take longer to heal than muscle pulls.

If you strain a muscle, apply ice as an immediate first aid treatment. Rest the injured area. Healing is affected by many factors—age, physical condition, and so on—so citing an "average" healing time could be misleading. If the condition of your strain does not improve in what you consider a reasonable time, consult a doctor.

INJURIES NEEDING PROFESSIONAL ATTENTION

More serious injuries that can be incurred from repeated jogging, jumping, and landing in an aerobics class are now described. These injuries usually require medical attention.

Shinsplints

Pain over the anterior aspect of the lower leg is generally called *shinsplints*. Shinsplints usually result from overuse of the muscle-tendon units. The major muscles of the lower leg are contained within fascia (tissue) envelopes. If there is swelling in the muscles, the arterial inflow and venous outflow to the muscles of that compartment can be impaired, causing a slow, activity-related pain in the involved compartment (8).

Several factors contribute to the development of shinsplints. One factor is an involuntary collapsing of the arch of the foot, which causes the muscles of the medial longitudinal arch, rather than its ligaments, to support the bones of the arch. Since the ligaments are intended to be the primary supporters, when the muscles are forced to assume that role, they become overfatigued, irritated, and inflamed.

Another factor is an imbalance of muscular strength on the front (anterior) and the back (posterior) aspect of the shinbone (the tibia) (27). Jogging or jumping on hard surfaces, improper landings from jumps, and improper shoes are also factors contributing to the development of shinsplints.

Sprain

More serious than a strain, a *sprain* is a sudden or violent twisting or wrenching of a joint, causing the ligaments to stretch or tear and often the blood vessels to rupture, with hemorrhage into the surrounding tissues. Symptoms of a sprain are swelling, inflammation, point tenderness, and discoloration. Ankle sprains are the most common in aerobic workouts. The most frequent is the *inversion sprain*, which results from unstable landings (6). The ligaments on the outside of the ankle joint are the weakest in the ankle and are most susceptible to injury incurred by rolling over on the outside of the ankle.

Plantar Fascitis

Plantar fascitis is a direct injury or strain of the plantar fascia, the ligamentous support of the arch of the foot. The injury causes chronic pain and inflames the foot, in particular, the heel. A radiating discomfort may also affect the longitudinal arch. Another cause of plantar fascitis is overuse by putting too much stress on the feet in relation to the amount of conditioning training and preparation.

Achilles Tendinitis

Inflammation of the Achilles tendon, the tendon of the heel, is common to running sports. *Achilles tendinitis* is often the result of a single episode of overuse. However, it can often be the result of a muscle imbalance of the lower leg.

Chondromalacia Patella (Runner's Knee)

Aerobic exercisers may experience a vague pain in the knees when running, leaping, or stair stepping (or walking or running up and down stairs). This pain is characteristic of *chondromalacia patella*, or runner's knee—an erosion of the cartilage covering the underside of the kneecap, or patella. Internal factors that affect chondromalacia are anatomical malalignment of the lower extremities:

Discrepancy in leg length

Abnormality in rotation of the hips

Bowlegs

Knock-knees

Flat feet

Musculature imbalance

The following external factors can also promote the problem:

Training errors, including abrupt changes in intensity, duration, or frequency

Improper footwear

Bad running surfaces; avoid exercising on cement floors (3)

Patellar Tendinitis (Jumper's Knee)

Repetitive jumping and landing activities can produce small scars in the patellar tendon, causing pain, tenderness, and inflammation directly below the kneecap. Often an aching in the knees apparent at the beginning of a workout disappears after warm-up. However, pain recurs when activity ceases. In a worsened condition, pain continues throughout a workout, and pressing on the tendon itself causes pain.

Stress Fracture

A *stress fracture* is a small fracture caused by repetitive jogging, jumping, and landing. In most cases, it occurs in the shins or the ball of the foot, involving one or both of the small sesamoid bones located in this area of the foot. The injury causes chronic pain and swelling.

SUMMARY

Any sort of injury can take time away from your aerobic training program. Use proper precautions and common sense in initiating your training. If you are injured, remember the simple steps of first aid treatment: rest, ice, compression, and elevation; apply the treatment immediately after injury occurs. Seek medical advice for injuries that persist.

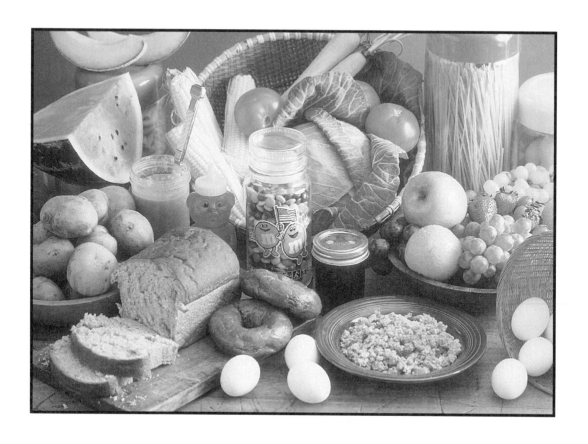

7

NUTRITION AND DIET

Nutrition is as important as regular exercise for staying in good health. The body cannot supply the strength and endurance needed for aerobic exercise if not properly fueled. The body's fuel is food, the source of energy to maintain life and perform work.

CALORIES

The energy food releases is measured in **calories,** or more specifically, **kilocalories.** The number of calories the body needs varies widely among individuals.

Virtually all the calories of energy the body uses are supplied by carbohydrates, fats, and proteins. Carbohydrates are the body's primary energy source. Fats are utilized if the carbohydrate supply is too low to meet the body's basic energy needs. Proteins provide an alternate energy source; the body uses them only when there are not enough calories available in the form of carbohydrates and fats. Protein is rarely used as an energy source; its most important function is to aid the body's growth and repair.

The amount of calories the body requires depends on the amount of calories (energy) it expends.

The energy output to maintain life functions—respiration, digestion, circulation and nerve, hormonal, and cellular activities—is called the **basal metabolic rate (BMR).** This is approximately $\frac{2}{3}$ of a person's energy use each day. Other energy output is for physical activities. The amount of energy you need each day depends on your age, size, and activity level. Energy is measured in calories, the fuel source for the body, and each and every food source has its own caloric value.

TABLE 7-1

CALORIC VALUES OF NUTRIENTS

Nutrient	Caloric Value
Protein	4 kilocalories per gram
Carbohydrate	4 kilocalories per gram
Fat	9 kilocalories per gram
Alcohol	7 kilocalories per gram

Not all foods are of equal caloric value. One food of equal weight to another can contain more calories just because of its value. Table 7-1 is a caloric value chart.

An example of how to determine the caloric value of food items is outlined below.

A piece of whole wheat bread that contains 2 grams of fat, 13 grams of carbohydrate, and 3 grams of protein would supply the following number of calories:

2 grams of fat = 18 calories

13 grams of carbohydrate = 52 calories

3 grams of protein = 12 calories

Caloric total = 80 calories

Approximately 23 percent fat

Approximately 64 percent carbohydrate

Approximately 13 percent protein

The type and combination of food fuel for the body is extremely important. We should all eat a well-balanced diet. Over the years, scientists and nutritionists have worked to define what "well-balanced" should be. A food guide was developed in 1950 and revised in 1978 to encourage people to eat a balanced selection of foods. This food guide, called the *Basic Four Food Group Plan,* includes the following four food groups:

1. Milk and milk products
2. Meats, fish, poultry, eggs, and substitutes of nuts and tofu and other soybean products
3. Fruits and vegetables
4. Breads and cereals

Since 1978, the Basic Four Food Group Plan has been modified to provide a better foundation for making food choices for a nutritionally adequate diet. The *Modified Basic Four Food Group Guide* includes

1. Milk and milk products
2. Protein foods
   Animal sources
   Legumes
   Nuts
3. Fruits and vegetables
   Vitamin C–rich
   Dark green
   Other
4. Whole-grain cereal products
5. Fats and oils

In 1992, the U.S. Department of Agriculture replaced the Basic Four Food Group Plan with a basic five-food group plan called the *Food Guide Pyramid.* In the pyramid, fruits and vegetables each have their own group. Fats, oils, and sweets are not considered a food group and are to be used sparingly. The food pyramid and the recommended servings of each food group are shown in Table 7-2. Using either the Modified Basic Four Food Guide or the Food Guide Pyramid can provide a guideline that is nutritionally sound in making choices of food selection.

NUTRIENTS

The food we eat is made up of nutrients. To fully understand the basics of proper nutrition, you should also become familiar with the types of nutrients that the body requires and their functions.

Protein

Protein is the basic structural substance of each cell in the body, and the main function of protein is to build and repair body tissue. Protein is

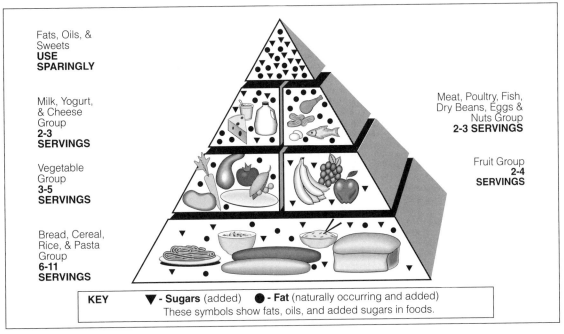

Fats, Oils, &
Sweets
**USE
SPARINGLY**

Milk, Yogurt,
& Cheese
Group
**2-3
SERVINGS**

Meat, Poultry, Fish,
Dry Beans, Eggs &
Nuts Group
2-3 SERVINGS

Vegetable
Group
**3-5
SERVINGS**

Fruit Group
**2-4
SERVINGS**

Bread, Cereal,
Rice, & Pasta
Group
**6-11
SERVINGS**

KEY   ▼ - **Sugars** (added)   ● - **Fat** (naturally occurring and added)
These symbols show fats, oils, and added sugars in foods.

TABLE 7-2   THE FOOD GUIDE PYRAMID

also required to make **hemoglobin,** which carries oxygen to the cells. Protein is essential for muscular contraction during activity and plays an important role in regulating body fluids in acid base quality during vigorous exercise. Protein is also required to form antibodies in the bloodstream to fight off infection and disease.

Protein is made of basic building blocks called *amino acids.* Of the 22 amino acids in protein, 8 are considered essential. These essential amino acids cannot be manufactured in the body and therefore must be supplied through the food we eat. The protein in animal food sources is called complete because it contains the eight essential amino acids. The animal food sources are meat, fish, poultry, eggs, milk, and milk products.

Plant protein sources cannot supply the necessary total protein source because they lack one or more of the essential amino acids. However, when properly combined, these incomplete plant protein sources can provide all eight essential amino acids. Plant protein food sources are lentils, legumes, nuts, cereal, and tofu or other soybean products.

A general guide to creating complete proteins by combining plant proteins is to combine animal proteins with grains or legumes, or different plant protein sources:

Animal Protein and Grains
• milk and cereal
• cheese pizza
• cheese and noodle casserole

Animal Protein and Legumes
• lentil soup and cheese toast
• chili with beans
• refried beans and cheese burrito

Plant and Plant Proteins
• beans and corn
• beans and rice
• beans and noodles
• black-eyed peas and rice

Tofu, a high-quality alternative to animal protein, is made from soymilk and is low in saturated fat and calories and free of cholesterol.

Protein intake should comprise approximately 12 percent of daily total calories. This means 6 to 9 ounces of protein per day, or 0.9 grams of protein per kilogram of body weight (multiply your body weight in pounds by 0.424 to obtain your weight in kilograms) (34). Pregnant and nursing mothers are exceptions to this protein requirement; they should increase their protein intake by 10 and 20 grams, respectively (29). Also an exception are individuals involved in strenuous power and strength-building programs. Protein intake for such athletes should be approximately 1.0–1.5 grams of protein per kilogram of body weight (15).

Many Americans eat an excess of protein, primarily animal protein. Although animal protein in a diet is a good way to ensure a balanced supply of essential amino acids, animal protein is high in saturated fats. Additionally, an excessive intake of protein can be stressful to the body in the process of breaking the protein down for fuel usage and for elimination. Most nutritionists recommend reducing the consumption of animal protein and increasing the intake of plant (vegetable) protein.

Fats

Dietary fats have the highest energy content of all nutrients. Fat's main function is to supply fuel and energy to the body, both at rest and during exercise. Fat also helps the body use the fat-soluble vitamins A, D, E, and K. Body fat also has other functions, such as cushioning the body's vital organs and protecting them from extreme temperatures of cold.

Although there is no specific requirement for fat in the diet, there is a need for essential fatty acid and the vitamins that are the components of fat. Currently, about 40 percent of Americans' daily caloric intake is composed of fat. A recommended dietary goal is less than 30 percent, with the amount of saturated fat in the diet less than 10 percent (35). In general, to maintain a healthy diet, the total amount of fats in the diet should be reduced; and saturated fats should be replaced with unsaturated fats.

When we are referring to fats we are really talking about **lipids.** The three lipids we are con-

cerned with are **triglycerides** (fats and oils), **phospholipids,** and **sterols.**

Triglycerides Triglycerides make up approximately 98 percent of our fat intake from food. All foods with fat contain a combination of saturated and unsaturated fats. The difference between saturated and unsaturated fatty acid molecules is that the carbon atoms are "saturated" with hydrogen atoms in saturated fats, whereas unsaturated fats may have only one or more double bonds between carbon and hydrogen atoms.

Saturated fats are found predominantly in animal meat, poultry fats, and animal products such as eggs and dairy items. Plant-saturated fats are found in coconut and palm oil, vegetable shortening, and commercial bakery pastries and sweets.

Unsaturated fats generally come from plant sources and are usually liquid at room temperature. If only one double bond of carbon and hydrogen is present, the fat is said to be monosaturated. Examples of monosaturated fats are canola, olive, and peanut oil. If two or more double bonds between carbon and hydrogen exist, the fat is said to be polyunsaturated. Polyunsaturated fats include safflower, sunflower, soybean, and corn oil.

A type of polyunsaturated fat belonging to the omega-3 family of fatty acids has recently been proposed to be a health benefit. This type of polyunsaturated fat is found in the fish and fish oil of cold-water fish such as tuna, herring, sardines, and mackerel. Including this fat in the diet seems to help prevent clots from forming on artery walls. Another polyunsaturated fatty acid, linoleic acid, found in cooking and salad oils, must be consumed in the diet and cannot be synthesized by the body. Linoleic acid is essential for growth, reproduction, skin maintenance, cell membranes, and general body functions (29).

Phospholipids Phospholipids are a combination of one or more fatty acid molecules with phosphoric acid and a nitrogen base. Phospholipids are important for blood clotting and are found in the structure of the insulation sheath of the nerve fibers. In the phospholipid family are lipoproteins, which transport fat in the blood. There are two types of lipoproteins: high-density lipoproteins and low-density lipoproteins.

Low-density lipoproteins (LDLs) have the least amount of protein and the greatest amount of fat. LDLs have the greatest amount of *cholesterol*, which is the fat in the blood and that found in tissues. Cholesterol is important to the production of hormones and enzymes but, when carried by the LDL, it has an affinity to deposit on the arterial wall. The continued buildup of cholesterol narrows the artery, increasing the chances of coronary heart disease.

High-density lipoproteins (HDLs) have the greatest amount of protein and the least amount of fat and cholesterol. HDLs protect against heart disease. They compete with the LDLs to enter into the cells of artery walls. HDLs carry cholesterol deposited on the artery wall to the liver and from there it is excreted by the intestines, thus combating the risk of coronary heart disease.

When a physician determines your cholesterol level, the amount of LDLs and HDLs can be determined. The ratio of these lipoproteins can help provide information in predicting the risk of coronary heart disease. The good news for people involved in an aerobics fitness program is that studies have shown that the HDL level can be increased with regular aerobic exercise.

Sterols The most widely known sterol is cholesterol. Cholesterol is found only in animal tissue that contains no fatty acids. Cholesterol is important in the production of hormones and enzymes and is also a part of cell membranes. Dietary cholesterol, which is the cholesterol found in animal products, raises the total level of blood cholesterol. When an excess of cholesterol is taken in the diet, it is deposited by the LDLs on the arterial walls. The highest amounts of cholesterol are found in liver and other organ meats and in egg yolks. To create a healthy diet and to lower the risk of coronary heart disease, dietary cholesterol should be reduced.

Carbohydrates

Carbohydrates supply the body with its primary source of energy, glucose. Glucose (blood sugar) is the product of the digestion of carbohydrates and is stored in the muscles. Carbohydrates also provide fuel for the central nervous system and are a metabolic primer for fat metabolism (29).

Although all carbohydrates have a certain chemistry in common, there is a big difference between one carbohydrate and another. The two general types of carbohydrates are simple and complex. **Simple carbohydrates** — sugars — are maltose, which is found in malt; lactose, found in milk; and sucrose, which is table sugar. When these sugars are ingested, they are converted to blood glucose almost immediately. Therefore, the consumption of simple carbohydrates causes blood glucose levels to fluctuate too quickly, making energy levels vacillate. Table sugar and the refined and processed sugars found in sodas, candy, cookies, cakes, and a realm of other sweetened treats offer no nutrients, are high in calories, and are associated with tooth decay, obesity, malnutrition, diabetes, and hypoglycemia (low blood sugar).

Complex carbohydrates — starches — are the natural sugars found in fruits, vegetables, and grains. They are the best source of energy because they convert blood glucose slowly. In other words, they supply a sustained energy output.

Complex carbohydrates are probably the best foods we can eat because they are high in vitamins, minerals, and fiber. Fiber is the structural part of fruits, vegetables, legumes, cereals, and grains that humans cannot break down in the digestive system. It provides the roughage and bulk to keep the gastrointestinal tract working properly. Fiber has been shown to lower cholesterol and help control diabetes, and it may also help prevent colon cancer.

Daily caloric intake should include about 60 percent carbohydrates, with about half of that intake being complex carbohydrates. You should make every effort to decrease your intake of simple, "sugary" carbohydrates, which have no nutritional value, and increase your intake of complex carbohydrates, which offer vitamins, minerals, and fiber.

Water

Water is second to oxygen as a substance necessary to sustain life. An adequate supply of water is necessary for all energy production in the body, for temperature control (especially during vigorous exercise), and for the elimination of waste products. *Dehydration,* or the loss of water in the body, can increase the risk of heat exhaustion and heatstroke. You should include water as an essential part of your diet and be sure to drink water, especially before and after exercise. When your teacher calls for a break during class, take the opportunity to get a drink from the water fountain or your water bottle. It is important to drink small amounts of water ($\frac{1}{2}$ to 1 cup) every 15 minutes during exercise.

Water taken prior to exercise should be approximately 1½ cups about 15 minutes before activity. After exercise, water taken should be 1 to 2 cups per pound lost during the workout due to water loss through sweating.

Although a number of commercial products claim to replenish the body by replacing not only fluids but also electrolytes and carbohydrates, these drinks contain sugar. Sugar slows the rate at which water leaves the stomach, thus delaying the rehydration process. The best way to replace fluid lost in exercise is with water; and cold water leaves the stomach more quickly than warm water, thus helping you to cool down more rapidly.

Drinking six to eight glasses of water a day is recommended for health maintenance. If you are physically active, you need to drink more than eight glasses and should follow the guidelines described earlier.

Alcohol

Alcohol remains as the most widely used drug on American college campuses and is a major problem even in high schools. Although alcohol is a drug, it is classified as a nutrient because it provides energy; one gram of alcohol is equal to 7 kilocalories. Although alcohol is classified as a nutrient, it adds no nutritional value to our diet. Alcohol is metabolized as a carbohydrate, stored mainly as a fat, and has adverse effects on athletic performance. The use of alcohol decreases aerobic capacity and strength. Alcohol decreases the liver's output of glucose, a prime ingredient for the production of ATP. The use of alcohol increases fatigue, promotes difficulty in regulating body temperature, and dehydrates the body. New research, published in the *Journal of the American Medical Association* (1994), notes that the consumption of one or two drinks a day has been associated with lowered heart attack mortality. However, consumption of three or more drinks a day has been linked to increased mortality from other causes. The general message is that alcohol consumption in excess may pose problems of fat accumulation and decrease in health.

Vitamins and Minerals

Vitamins help utilize and absorb other nutrients and are necessary for the body's normal metabolic functioning. Vitamins are classified as fat soluble or water soluble. *Fat-soluble vitamins* (A, D, E, and K) tend to remain stored in the body and are usually not excreted in the urine. An excess accumulation of these vitamins may be toxic to the body. *Water-soluble vitamins* (C and B complex) are excreted in the urine and are not stored in the body in appreciable amounts.

Minerals are the building materials for body tissues and serve as nerve regulators. Minerals, except iron, are excreted by the body after they have carried out the function they provide for the body. Because minerals are excreted, it is important to regularly replace mineral losses.

Vitamins and minerals work together to regulate body processes, releasing energy from food and helping to metabolize carbohydrates and fats. Although there is a growing concern regarding vitamin deficiency, most people, except for unusual cases, can easily obtain the required amount of vitamins and minerals through good nutritional habits. Table 7-3 provides a list of the major vitamins and minerals, their functions, and food sources. Table 7-4 summarizes the four parts of balanced meals. Table 7-5 is an outline of food sources for planning a well-balanced, nutritionally sound diet throughout the year.

In addition to being aware of eating a diet that provides the necessary vitamins and minerals, you should also take heed of certain nutrient combinations. For instance, don't take calcium with an iron supplement or with a multiple vitamin that contains iron, because iron impairs the body's uptake of the calcium. Iron taken in the form of ferrous sulfate can destroy vitamin E. Beware of foods that rob the body of key nutrients, impairing the absorption of particular vitamins and minerals. Caffeine, found not only in coffee but also in many soft drinks, causes a loss of vitamin B1, calcium, and iron. Hot dogs, bacon, and lunch meats that contain nitrates rob the body of vitamin A. With alcohol, the body loses vitamins B1, B6, B12, and D. Medication can also rob the body of key nutrients. With antibiotics and birth control pills, the body loses vitamin B complex. Aspirin impairs the absorption of calcium, zinc, magnesium, iron, and vitamin B complex. Last but not least, our emotions also affect our body's ability to fully retain our vitamins and minerals. Stress, something, that unfortunately we all experience, robs the body of vitamins B3, B12, and C as well as calcium and zinc.

WEIGHT LOSS: THE "SET-POINT" THEORY

If weight loss were merely a reflection of decreasing total caloric intake by diet, it would certainly be a simple matter to lose weight. Although weight loss normally occurs at the onset of a diet, the body's weight tends to stabilize at some new, lower level. To continue to lose weight becomes difficult. Long-term weight control is explained by new insights of weight control in the set-point theory.

The set-point theory maintains that the brain's hypothalamus regulates weight by comparing the body's current level of fat with a kind of constant internal standard. When a person's fat level falls below this internal standard, the body responds with increased appetite. If food intake is not increased, the body adjusts its metabolic rate to protect its usual level of fat stores. During a diet, when food intake is not increased to meet the body's increased appetite demands, the body adjusts its metabolic rate by burning calories more slowly. When a dieter resumes normal eating patterns, it is not uncommon to experience weight regain due to the body's slower metabolic rate.

The body's slower metabolic rate also affects the total fat-burning capacity of the body. The slowdown of the body's fat-burning capacity is due partly to a decrease in lean body mass, or muscle. During dieting, much of the weight loss occurs from the fat that is burned in muscle tissue. Finally, dieting causes enzyme changes in the adipose tissue lipoprotein lipase (a fat-storing enzyme). When caloric intake is decreased, this enzyme is dramatically increased, causing the body to become more efficient at storing fat.

Rather than attempting to lose weight through dieting, the set-point theory maintains that to lose weight, the body's set point must be lowered. The most effective way to lower the set point is through exercise. Once the set point is lowered, the body will work to maintain the lower fat level, just as it tried to maintain the higher fat level described in the dieting process. As opposed to dieting, weight loss through exercise maintains muscle mass. Remember that most fat is burned within the muscle. Through exercise, fat is lost; thus the ratio of muscle to fat is increased. The increased ratio of muscle to fat also has long-term benefits since muscle requires more calories than fat to maintain itself.

Exercise also changes the enzymes of the muscle system to be more effective in burning fat. Oxidative enzymes are increased as a result of moderate aerobic exercise, thus increasing

TABLE 7-3

VITAMIN AND MINERAL FUNCTIONS AND FOOD SOURCES

Vitamin	Function	Source
A	Enhances quality of skin, clear vision; helps maintain strong teeth.	Fortified milk, carrots, pumpkins, sweet potatoes, squash, and green vegetables
B Complex Folic Acid	Prevents anemia, certain birth defects of the spine and brain; helps make DNA. Works best when combined with B12. Oral contraceptives may increase need for folic acid.	Dark green and leafy vegetables, enriched cereals and legumes
B6 Pyrodoxine	For energy production and red blood cell formation.	Avocados, baked potatoes, and leafy green vegetables
B12 Cobalamin	Maintains red blood cells and functions of the nervous system. If B12 is low, aerobic capacity seems to diminish and you may experience difficulty with balance and coordination. Stress and medications can impair absorption. Vegetarians who do not eat meat, eggs, or dairy products can be at risk of B12 deficiency.	Raw oysters, raw clams, sardines canned in soybean oil, fish, liverwurst, creamed cottage cheese, milk, and eggs
C	Helps make oxygen-carrying red blood cells and hemoglobin, which are important for bones and teeth.	Citrus fruits, tomatoes, strawberries, green and red peppers, potatoes, cranberries, pineapples, and orange juice
D	Promotes bone growth and strength.	Fortified milk, egg yolk, tuna, salmon, cod liver oil, and liver (Liver intake should be monitored due to high cholesterol level.)
E	For red blood cell formation.	Fortified cereals, nuts, seeds, and oils. avocado, mango, spinach, sweet potato, and wild rice •
K	For bone metabolism and blood clotting. Reduces risk and severity of bone fractures. K in combination with calcium, magnesium, and boron is called the "bone formula."	Leafy green vegetables, cabbage, peas, cauliflower, kale, broccoli, watercress, and dried beans

the ability of the muscles to burn fat and to lose fat stores.

With respect to the set-point theory, the type of exercise for weight control is crucial. Aerobic exercise is the most beneficial because it allows the body to burn fat effectively during exercise.

To achieve weight loss, aerobic exercise must be done at a moderate pace and at least 5 days a week. Although research indicates that 3 days a week yields an aerobic effect, 4 days a week appears to be the threshold for weight loss, while 6 to 7 days a week seems to be the ideal.

Mineral	Function	Source
Calcium	Strengthens bones and teeth; essential for cell function, muscle contraction, blood clotting, and transmission of nerve impulses.	Dairy products, broccoli, salmon, sardines, tofu, kale, spinach, and almond
Iron	Formation of hemoglobin and myoglobin, which aids in the storage and transport of oxygen within cells. Is depleted with exercise due to sweating. Diets low in iron may lead to anemia.	Organ meats, egg yolk, fish, oysters, milk, legumes, apricots, dried fruits, whole grain cereals, greens, broccoli, and molasses
Magnesium	Facilitates intestine absorption of calcium; required for teeth and bone formation, muscle contraction, transmission of nerve impulses.	Chocolate, instant coffee, cashews, and artichokes
Potassium	In combination with sodium and calcium, maintains normal heart rhythm, regulates body's water balance, aids in muscle contraction, and conducts nerve impulses.	Potatoes, legumes, citrus fruits, bananas, tomatoes, and leafy vegetables
Zinc	Aids in wound healing and promotes mental alertness; necessary for stress and tissue repair. Intense exercise can decrease the body's zinc stores due to sweating.	Oysters, legumes, brewer's yeast, meat, whole-grain cereals, cashews, sunflower and pumpkin seeds, and tofu

WEIGHT LOSS FALLACIES

Fad Diets

Weight loss programs are promoted by every avenue of media possible. Promises of simple and easy methods of weight loss and body toning are weekly features. Avoid fad diets, many of which can produce hazardous health problems. Never eliminate calories totally from one food group, as is called for in many fad diets. If you lose weight quickly, your body does not

TABLE 7-4

PLANNING BALANCED MEALS
BALANCED MEALS HAVE FOUR PARTS

Nutrient	Food	Why?
1. Fiber	vegetables fruits	• Swells like a sponge in your stomach keeping you full longer • Helps regulate cholesterol level in your blood • Helps keep blood sugar at proper levels
2. Complex Carbohydrate	vegetables fruits cereals pasta starchy vegetables crackers and snacks	• Provides constant energy for your brain • Provides complementary source of protein for meatless meals • Helps keep blood sugar at proper levels
3. Protein	beans nuts seeds dairy products eggs meat fish	• Keeps food in stomach so you feel full longer • Builds and repairs muscles • Provides complementary source of protein for meatless meals • Helps keep blood sugar at proper levels
4. Fat*	avocado oils margarine mayonnaise salad dressing animal fats cream cheese	• Keeps food in stomach so you feel full longer • Provides vitamin E and essential fatty acids • Helps keep blood sugar at proper levels

*Note: Small quantities of fat can usually be included at every meal for diets providing 30% of calories from fat. For diets providing less than 30% of calories from fat, it may be not be possible to include fat at every meal.

© 1994 Dietitian's Weight Control Program, Inc.

have enough time to adapt to the lower calorie intake, so you usually gain back the lost weight. And diets that promote quick weight loss by the elimination of water cause dehydration and the loss of important minerals (24).

Weight Loss Products

Avoid also being fooled by products that produce weight loss through dehydration such as plastic/rubber garments, body wraps, or saunas and steambaths. It is extremely important to avoid weight loss programs that use diet pills that are addictive and may cause health problems such as increased blood pressure, irregular heartbeat, and insomnia. The effect of a suppressed appetite from the use of diet pills is temporary, because the body builds up a tolerance to these stimulants.

TABLE 7-5
SEASONAL FOOD SHOPPING GUIDE

January	*February*	*March*	*April*	*May*	*June*
Apple*	Apple*	Apple*	Apple*	Cantaloupe*	Apricot*
Grapefruit	Grapefruit	Grapefruit	Grapefruit	Cherry	Berries
Orange	Orange	Orange	Mango*	Mango*	Cantaloupe*
Tangelo	Strawberry	Pineapple	Orange	Orange	Cherry
Tangerine		Strawberry	Pineapple	Pineapple	Honeydew*
	Broccoli		Strawberry	Strawberry	Lime
Avocado*	Brussels	Artichoke			Mango*
Broccoli	Sprouts	Asparagus	Artichoke	Artichoke	Nectarine*
Brussels Sprouts	Cauliflower	Avocado*	Asparagus	Asparagus	Peach*
Cauliflower	Green Pea	Broccoli	Avocado*	Avocado*	Pineapple
Spinach	Spinach	Cauliflower	Bean	Bean	Plum*
Sweet Potato	Sweet Potato	Green Pea	Broccoli	Broccoli	Prune
		Radish	Cauliflower	Cauliflower	Watermelon*
July	*August*	Spinach	Green Pea	Green Pea	
		Sweet Potato	Radish	Radish/	Asparagus
Apricot*	Berries		Spinach	Spinach	Avocado*
Berries	Cantaloupe*	*September*	Sweet Potato	Sweet Potato	Bean
Cantaloupe*	Cherry				Beet
Cherry	Grape	Apple*	*October*	*November*	Bell Pepper
Grape	Honeydew*	Coconut			Corn
Honeydew*	Lime	Cranberry	Apple*	Apple*	Cucumber
Lime	Mango*	Grape	Coconut	Coconut	Green Pea
Mango*	Nectarine*	Melons*	Cranberry	Cranberry	Radish
Nectarine*	Peach*	Nectarine*	Grape	Grape	Squash (Summer)
Papaya*	Plum*	Peach*	Honeydew*	Grapefruit	Tomato
Peach*	Prune	Pear*	Nectarine*	Kiwi (California)	
Plum*	Watermelon*	Plum*	Pear*	Pear*	*December*
Prune		Pomegranate	Persimmon	Persimmon	
Watermelon*	Bean	Prune	Pomegranate	Pomegranate	Apple*
	Beet		Tangelo	Tangelo	Coconut
Bean	Bell Pepper	Avocado*		Tangerine	Cranberry
Beet	Corn	Bean	Avocado*		Grapefruit
Bell Pepper	Cucumber	Beet	Bell Pepper	Avocado*	Kiwi (California)
Corn	Okra	Bell Pepper	Brussels Sprouts	Broccoli	Orange
Cucumber	Squash	Cauliflower	Cauliflower	Brussels Sprouts	Persimmon
Green Pea	(Summer)	Corn	Corn	Cauliflower	Tangelo
Okra	Tomato*	Cucumber	Cucumber	Squash (Winter,	Tangerine
Radish		Eggplant	Eggplant	Pumpkin)	
Squash (Summer)		Okra	Squash (Winter,	Sweet Potato	Avocado*
Tomato*		Squash	Pumpkin(	Tomato*	Broccoli
		(Summer)	Sweet Potato		Brussels Sprouts
		Sweet Potato	Tomato*		Cauliflower
		Tomato*			Sweet Potato

Ripens at room temperature. Always in season: banana, cabbage, celery, lettuce, mushroom, onion, potato.

© 1994 Dietitian's Weight Control Program, Inc.

Is It Possible to Spot Reduce?

Evidence proves that spot reducing is a claim, *not* a fact. The public has been led to believe that blubbery thighs, hips, and arms are merely cosmetic problems. People who promote spot reducing are actually reinforcing a sedentary lifestyle, which is an initial factor in bringing about weight gain and muscular degeneration in the first place.

Exercise of a particular muscle cannot decrease the number of fat cells that lie immediately around that muscle. Also, exercise does not change fat into muscle; fatty tissue and muscular tissue are *not* the same and are not interchangeable. The only way to rid your body of unsightly fat is to reduce the amount of fat or to reduce the size of existing fat tissues.

Working muscles draw their source of energy from fat all over the body. As a result of exercise, fat from all over the body is released, converted into energy, and then used by the muscles. This breakdown of fat to energy is due to the interaction of the nervous, circulatory, muscular, and endocrine systems and is the only way to rid the body of its fatty deposits.

Spot-reducing exercises *seem* to work for two reasons. First, we tend to lose fat first from the area of greatest concentration. Second, when normally unexercised, weakened muscles are exercised, the muscle beneath the fat tissue is strengthened and toned. For example, a woman plagued with what appears to be fat deposits on the back of her arm may really have a weakened triceps muscle. Push-ups and arm-strengthening exercises can help strengthen and tone that muscle, firming the arm area. The circumference of that area may be reduced as a result of improved muscle tone. As a consequence, it may appear that the spot-reducing exercise works.

But do not be fooled; fat cannot be rolled, shimmied, or shaken off. Saunas and rubberized sweat suits won't rid you of pounds of fat—only water! Only a comprehensive fitness program can help you evaluate your fitness and fat level and help you achieve better overall health and fitness.

EATING DISORDERS

Anorexia nervosa is an eating disorder that involves severe food restriction as a means to weight loss. People who suffer from this disorder are usually very preoccupied with thinness and body image. They may often be involved seriously with a sport such as gymnastics or ballet that requires low body weight or an activity such as modeling. A person suffering from anorexia may be recognized by a severe loss of weight. But anorexia may cause other health problems, such as retarded bone growth, anemia, low blood pressure, amenorrhea, low body temperature, low basal metabolism, slow heart rate, and other physiological body changes. Anorexia should be treated by a qualified professional.

Bulimia is an eating disorder that involves episodes of excessive eating usually followed by purging. Binge eating usually involves eating high-calorie foods, generally sweets; eating during a time when no one can witness food consumption; ending a binge because of abdominal pain or with vomiting or by sleeping. A person who binge eats usually makes repeated attempts to lose weight, sometimes through excessive exercise, and there are visible signs of frequent weight fluctuations. A bulimic may feel guilty, shameful, and out of control and has low self-esteem. Binge eating can also produce a variety of health problems. Excessive eating can cause problems to the gastrointestinal tract, while the vomiting following the binge eating may cause an electrolyte imbalance and damage the enamel of the teeth. Bulimia should be treated by a qualified professional, and psychotherapy is usually recommended to help with the feelings of low self-esteem associated with this disorder.

SUCCESS IN WEIGHT CONTROL

Success in weight control depends upon being able to choose a program that will lead to life-long, sound nutritional habits. A diet should include foods that are affordable, easy to buy and prepare, and tasty. The caloric value of the foods should provide a weight loss of no more than 1 to 2 pounds per week. It is important to avoid programs that will cause weight loss too quickly with an end result of regaining the lost weight. The main idea is to lose weight and maintain the weight loss. A weight control program should include a form of aerobic exercise a minimum of 3 days a week. Ideally, 5–7 days a week of aerobic exercise is recommended for weight loss. However, if the person is beginning a new program from a sedentary state, it is advisable to begin a program and gradually increase the frequency of exercise periods.

Finally, bear in mind that we all have good intentions of eating a nutritionally balanced diet. But even with the best intentions, life's unexpected challenges — busy schedules, trying to lose weight, illness, and stress — can keep you from getting all the proper and necessary nutrition. You may want to consult a registered dietitian, sports medicine nutritionist, or physician to evaluate your diet. Most importantly, try to pay a little more attention to what it is you are eating on a regular or daily basis. At the end of this book is a worksheet designed to increase your awareness of your daily eating patterns and to help you achieve improved nutritional habits. Also use Tables 7-1 through 7-4 to help you achieve your nutritional goals.

Remember that a weight control program should ultimately provide new eating and exercise habits that can be sustained for life.

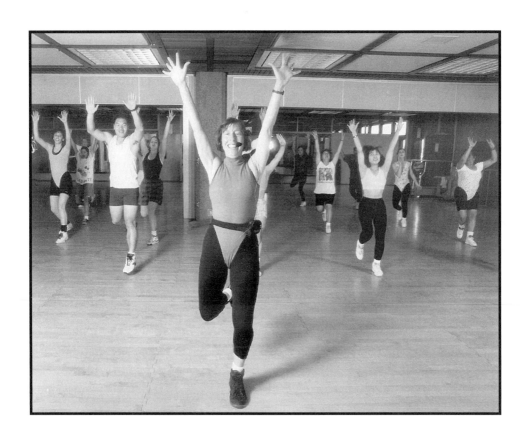

8

FLOOR AEROBIC MOVEMENTS

Floor aerobic movements are drawn from many areas of fitness. The steps can be pedestrian moves, dance moves, and athletic moves. The main goal of the movements used during the aerobic phase of the class is that, performed nonstop for a minimum of 20 minutes, they are intense enough to sustain an individual's target heart rate. You must pace yourself during the entire workout so that you are able to complete the aerobic section. If you find yourself tiring at any time, decrease the intensity of the moves. Never come to a complete stop. Reminder: Carefully monitor your heart rate by taking your pulse 5 minutes into the aerobic phase. Repeat this procedure at the middle and end of the aerobic workout.

This chapter describes the movements commonly used in the aerobic phase of the class, dis-

cusses combinations of these movements, and outlines precautions to follow in the aerobic class. A discussion of how to choreograph aerobic routines, and examples of routines for the various phases of the aerobics class are also included.

WHEN TO USE THESE MOVEMENTS

All of the movements that will be described can be used for the active warm-up at the beginning of the class—the aerobic warm-up that starts the aerobic phase—the peak aerobic section, and finally, the aerobic cool-down. The phase of the class will determine the intensity level at which you perform the movements. You can lower the intensity of any of the movements by

1. Lowering the arm positions
2. Lowering the height of the leg on any kicks or bends
3. Making the steps smaller
4. Changing any running movement into a walk
5. Deleting any jumps or hops and making them marches

You can increase the intensity of any low-impact movements by reversing these recommendations.

LOCOMOTOR MOVEMENTS

Locomotor movements are any movements that travel through space. Locomotor movements use the large muscles and are excellent for raising the heart rate. Because you are moving, you also lessen the impact on the body. It is important to use good technique when performing these movements; that is, land with the knees in a bent position and roll through your feet on all the landings.

Walking

A walk is a transfer of weight from one foot to the other, with one foot always on the ground.

Variations
Walking in place
Walking forward
Walking backward
Walking diagonally
Walking in a circle
Turning
Walking on your toes
Walking forward, stepping together; walking backward, stepping together; walking sideways, stepping together
Walking in a square

GRAPEVINE

1. Step to the left with your left foot.
2. Step to the left with your right foot crossing behind your left foot.
3. Step to the left with your left foot.
4. Step to the left with your right foot crossing in front of your left foot.

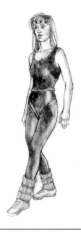
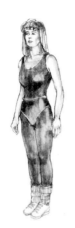

Walking backward, stepping together

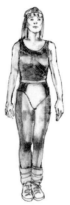

Stepping together

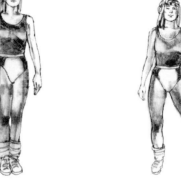

Walking sideways, left foot to side

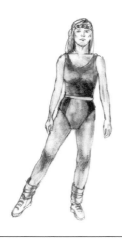

Walking sideways, right foot to side

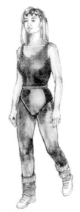
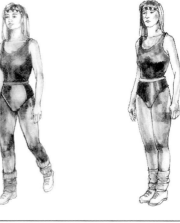

Walking forward, stepping together

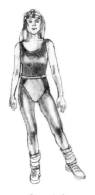
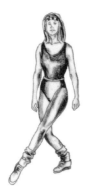

Step left   Cross behind

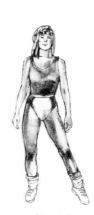
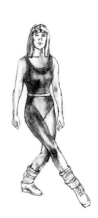

Step left   Cross front

Grapevine

> **PRECAUTION**
>
> *If the floor surface is uneven or car-*
> *peted, avoid lateral, or side-to-side,*
> *movements since these can be stressful*
> *to your knees and ankles.*

Running

A run is a transfer of weight from one foot to
the other. At one point in a run, both feet are off
the ground. A run is faster than a walk.

Variations
Running in place
Running forward
Running backward
Running diagonally
Running in a circle
Running in a figure eight
High-knee runs

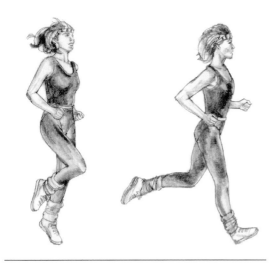

Running in place   Running forward

SCISSORS JUMPING JACKS

1. Jump with your feet together.
2. Jump with your legs splitting front and back; swing your arms in opposition.
3. Jump with your feet together; bring your arms to your sides.
4. Alternate legs on the split jump.

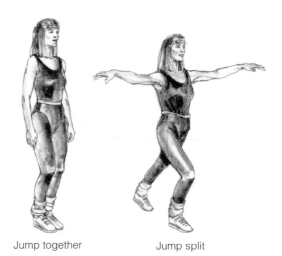

Jump together   Jump split

PRECAUTIONS

- *When running forward, run with your knees lifted and land with your heel first to put less stress on the calf muscles. Follow through by rolling onto the ball of your foot.*
- *When running in place, run with your knees lifted and land with the ball of your foot first. Follow through by pressing your heel to the floor.*

Jumping

A jump is an aerial movement in which a person takes off from two feet and lands on two feet.

Variations
Jumping in place
Jumping forward
Jumping backward
Jumping sideways
Jumping diagonally
Quarter, half, and whole turns

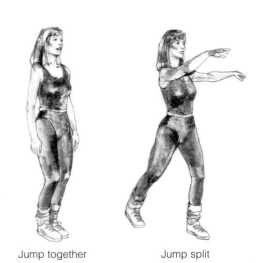

Jump together   Jump split

Scissors jumping jacks

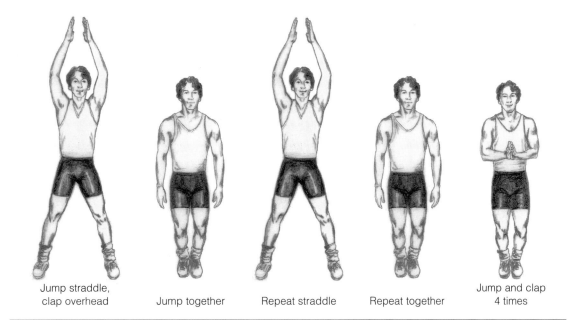

Jump straddle, clap overhead   Jump together   Repeat straddle   Repeat together   Jump and clap 4 times

Rhythm jacks

RHYTHM JACKS

1. Jump to a straddle position; clap your hands overhead.
2. Jump with your feet together; bring your arms down to your sides.
3. Jump to a straddle position; clap your hands overhead.
4. Jump with your feet together; bring your arms down to your sides.
5. Jump in place with your feet together four times, clapping on each jump.

MOVEMENT TIP

In rhythm jacks, clap your hands overhead or raise your arms to shoulder height.

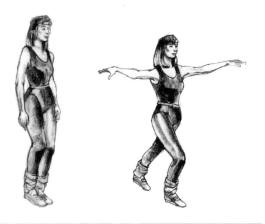

Jump lunge forward or backward

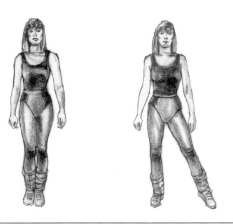

Jump lunge sideways

JUMP LUNGE

Alternately jump in place and then jump to a lunge position forward, backward, or sideways.

BREAKAWAY OR HEEL JACKS

1. Jump with your feet together; clap your hands.
2. Jump, extending one leg to the side, touching the heel of your extended leg to the floor; push your arm on the same side as the extended leg straight out to the side, and bend your other arm at the elbow at shoulder height.
3. Jump, your feet together, and repeat the exercise on your other side.

PRECAUTION

Always land from a jump with your knees bent. Land on the balls of your feet and press your heels down to make complete contact with the floor to absorb the shock of the jump, to avoid placing stress on the knees, and to stretch the Achilles tendons.

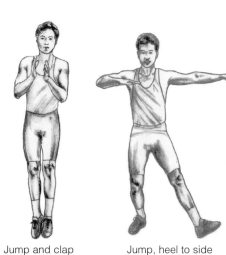

Jump and clap   Jump, heel to side

Breakaway or heel jacks

Hopping

A hop is an aerial movement in which a person takes off on one foot and lands on that same foot.

Variations

Hopping in place

Hopping forward

Hopping backward

Hopping diagonally

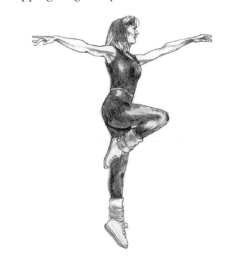

Hopping

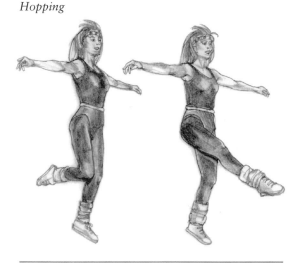

Hop-kick

HOP-KICK

Bend your lifted leg in and then kick to the front or side.

FLEA-HOP

1. Hop on one leg, lifting the opposite knee to hip height; swing arms in opposition.
2. Repeat this hop, alternating legs.

PENDULUM HOP

1. Hop on one leg, extending your other leg to the side at a 45-degree angle.
2. Repeat this hop, alternating legs.

MOVEMENT TIP

Pendulum hops may be performed as double hops or single hops or a combination of both.

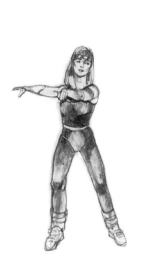 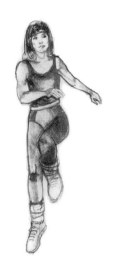 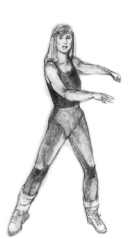 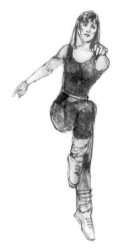

Step side   Hop with knee bend   Step on lifted leg   Hop with opposite knee bend

Flea-hop

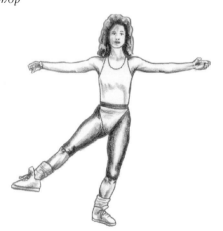 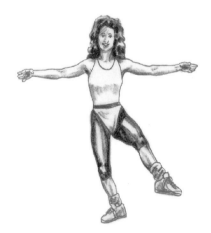

Pendulum hop

Leaping

A leap is an aerial movement in which a person moves from one foot to the other. Between the takeoff and landing, the body is suspended in air.

Variations

Leaping forward

Leaping backward

Leaping sideways

Leaping diagonally

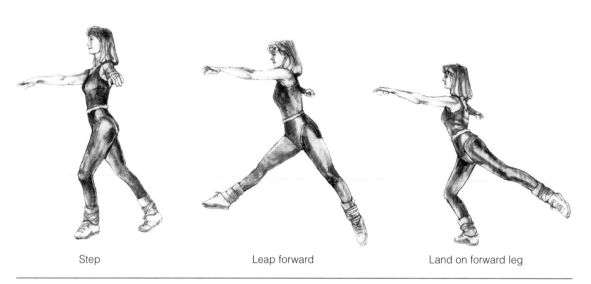

| Step | Leap forward | Land on forward leg |

Leaping

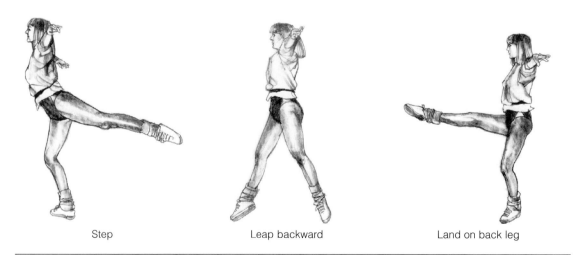

| Step | Leap backward | Land on back leg |

Leaping backward

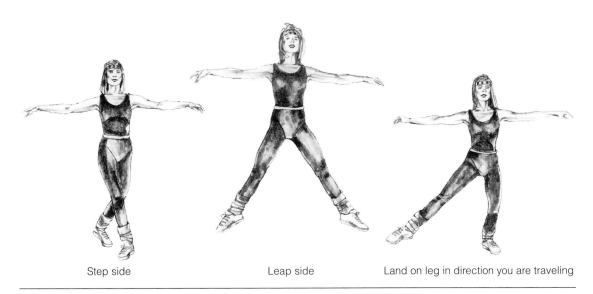

| Step side | Leap side | Land on leg in direction you are traveling |

Leaping sideways

Skipping

A skip is a combination of a step and a hop on the same foot, with an uneven rhythmic pattern.

Variations

Skipping forward

Skipping backward

Skipping sideways

Skipping in a circle

Turning

Sliding

A slide, or chassé, is a smooth, gliding, step-together-step. At its peak, the body is suspended in the air, with the legs together and fully extended.

Variations

Sliding forward

Sliding backward

Sliding sideways

AXIAL MOVEMENTS

Axial movements are any movements performed in one spot. You do not travel when you do these movements, although many of them

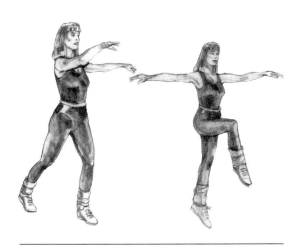

Skipping

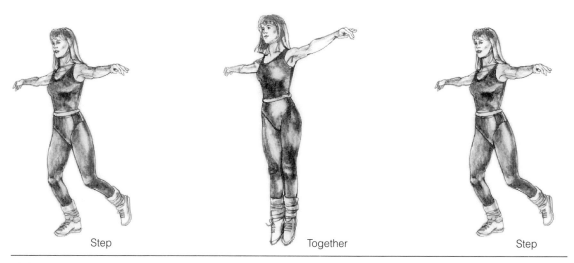

| Step | Together | Step |

Sliding

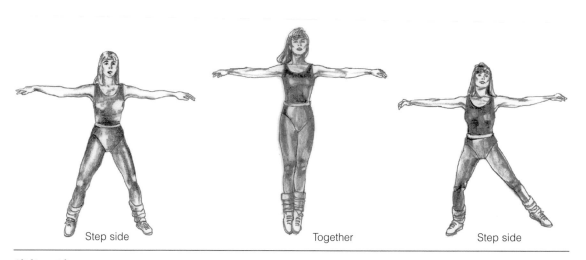

| Step side | Together | Step side |

Sliding sideways

can be done traveling forward, backward, or to the side. To lower intensity, you can perform these moves in one spot and without any jumping. To increase the intensity, add travel and jumping.

KNEE LIFTS

Perform to the front, back, or side.

KICKS

Perform to the front or to the side.

LUNGES

A lunge is a movement where the weight is on the front leg and that knee is bent. The other leg is extended to the floor either diagonally or to the side or to the back. You can alternate lunge legs, or you can do a number of repetitions on one leg before transferring to the other leg. Traveling lunges would alternate the lead leg—the

back leg would close and the opposite leg would go forward. This movement can be performed all the way across the room.

SQUATS

Although this movement is considered a calisthenic move, it is often used in the aerobic section. Start with the feet together and then open one leg about shoulder width apart and bend down as if you were sitting in a chair. Close the leg back to the starting position. Like the lunge, this movement can travel by closing the opposite foot to the starting position. You can also vary the intensity by jumping back to the starting position. You can perform the squat with the feet in a parallel position or a turned-out position.

JUMPING JACKS

A jumping jack starts with the feet together, and then you jump so that the feet land shoulder width apart. You then jump back to the starting position. Many variations exist (see section on jumping for variations).

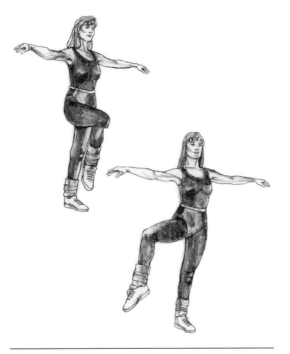

Knee lifts

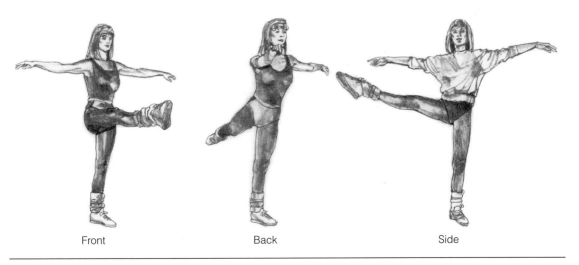

Front   Back   Side

Kicks

DANCE STEPS

KICK-BALL-CHANGE

Kick one leg to the front; then step to the rear of your supporting leg, placing your weight on the ball of your foot, with your heel lifted. Your other foot then steps in place, with your weight transferring onto this foot.

JAZZ SQUARE

The jazz square consists of four walking steps performed in a square pattern. Step forward with your right foot. Cross your left foot in front of your right. Step back on your right foot. Step to the left with your left foot. This step can start on either foot.

PIVOT TURN

Perform the pivot on two feet, quickly shifting your body to face in the opposite direction. Both of your feet remain on the floor in their positions as you pivot your body.

PADDLE TURN

The paddle turn is a simple turn that pivots your body around on one spot. Your weight shifts from one foot to the other. Your supporting, stationary leg pivots on the ball of the foot, with your heel lifting slightly off the floor. Your other leg extends to the side and "paddles" on the ball of the foot, rotating your body in a circular direction while your foot traces an imaginary circular pattern on the floor.

THREE-STEP TURN

Begin by stepping to the side. Step and rotate 180 degrees to face the back. Step and rotate 180 degrees to face the front. End the turn by bringing your feet together or touching the final stepping foot to the other foot.

MOVEMENT TIP

To get exact quarter turns, imagine a clock on the floor. Your "paddle" foot must touch at twelve o'clock, three o'clock, six o'clock, and nine o'clock.

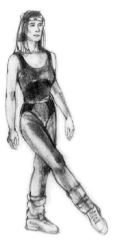
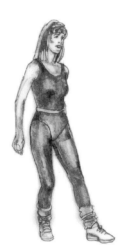
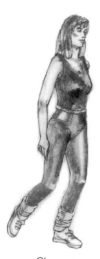

Kick   Ball   Change

Kick-ball-change

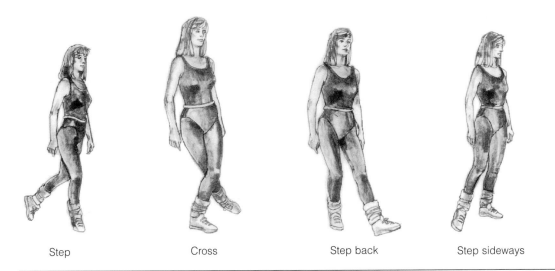

| Step | Cross | Step back | Step sideways |

Jazz square

MAMBO

This is a rocking step. Step forward on the right foot, then step back on the left foot. Step back on the right foot, then step forward on the left foot. You need to alternate the lead leg. Very often three quick steps are inserted at the last mambo in order to make this change.

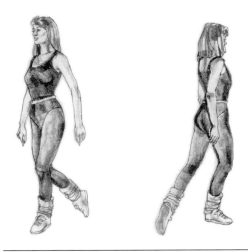

Pivot turn

CHA-CHA

The cha-cha is a combination of two slow steps, two quick steps, and a final slow step. The rhythm is 1-2-3 and 4. Step forward onto the full foot with your knees bent. Step back onto the ball of your opposite foot. On the triple "cha-cha-cha" steps, keep your knees bent and sway your hips, stepping in place or traveling very little. In floor aerobics, the cha-cha is modified with large step movements and traveling patterns.

CHARLESTON

Step forward onto your right foot. Swing your left leg forward to touch the floor, with the ball of your left foot ahead of your right foot. Step backward with your left foot. Swing your right leg back to touch the floor with the ball of your right foot behind your left foot. You may kick your leg instead of touching your foot to the floor to increase the intensity of the movement.

PONY

The pony is a combination of a small sideways leap and a ball change. Leap sideways right onto your right foot. Step onto the ball of your left foot. Quickly shift your body weight by stepping onto your right foot (change). Reverse the pony by leaping from your right foot to your left foot. The pony is done with bouncy stepping movements to increase intensity and a variety of foot patterns with the ball-change to add interest and variety.

ARM MOVEMENTS

You can perform variations of the basic movements by applying arm patterns. Those commonly used in aerobic dance include

Bow and arrow—keeping the arms at shoulder height, extend one arm to the side

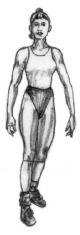
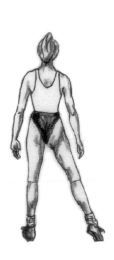
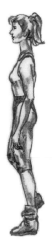
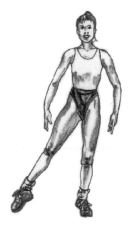

Paddle front   Paddle side   Paddle back   Paddle side

Paddle turn

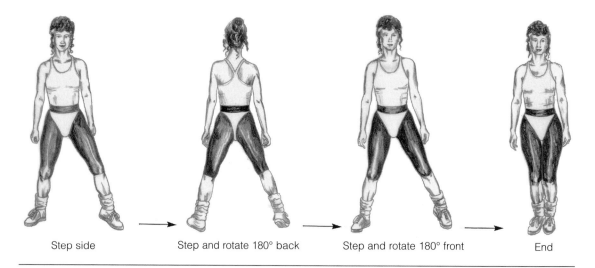

Step side   Step and rotate 180° back   Step and rotate 180° front   End

Three-step turn

and pull the other arm back at the elbow so that the fist ends by the shoulder. Alternate arms.

Arm circles—make small or large circles with your arms extended to the side and at shoulder height.

Arm scissors—alternately cross your straight arms in front or in back of your body.

Arm reaches—reach up, to the side, or down or do a combination of all three movements.

Karate punches—punch each of your arms diagonally across your body.

Pectoral press—hold your arms out to the side and bent upward from your elbows. Bring your forearms together in front of your face, elbows and wrists touching. Open your arms to the starting position.

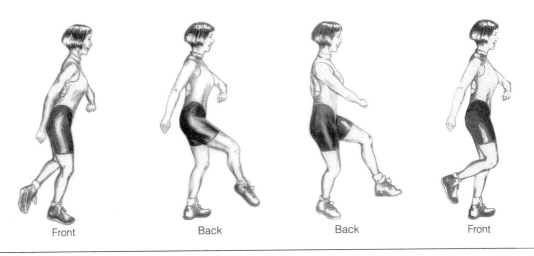

Front   Back   Back   Front

Mambo

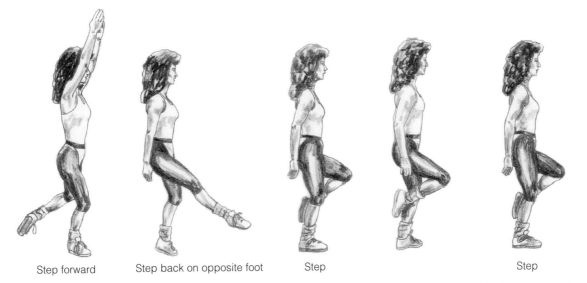

Step forward   Step back on opposite foot   Step   Step

Cha-cha

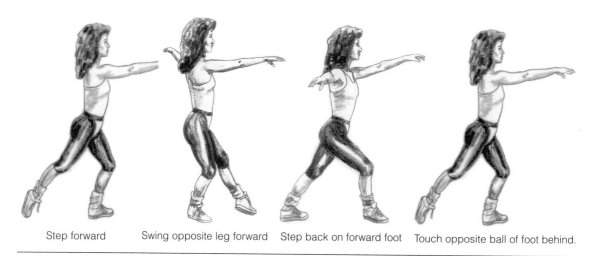

Step forward   Swing opposite leg forward   Step back on forward foot   Touch opposite ball of foot behind.

Charleston

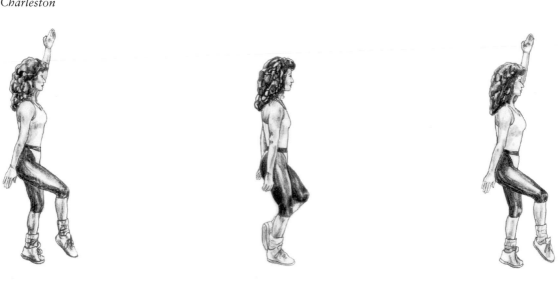

Pony

Coordination arms—stretch your arms straight out in front of your chest. Open your arms out to the side. Close your arms at chest height. Drop your arms straight down to slap the top of your thighs. This is a four-count movement.

Latin roll—keeping your arms bent at the elbows, roll your forearms in a circular

fashion around one another. Vary the roll at chest level, waist level, and above the head.

PRECAUTION

Avoid arm movements that violently fling your arms beyond the line of your shoulders, causing the chest muscles to overstretch.

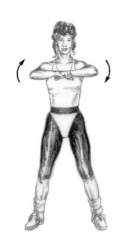

Latin roll

You can also use any of the arm movements described in Chapter 10. When choreographing arm patterns, it is helpful to vary the muscle groups that are used. By consulting Chapter 10, you can get a balanced upper-body workout along with your aerobic workout! Pay particular attention to excessive overhead arm movements, especially excessive lifting of the shoulder. These actions should be avoided!

COMBINATIONS OF MOVEMENTS

Just as the locomotor, axial, and dance step movements are endless, so too are the combinations of these movements. Listed are a few simple combinations derived from the steps already described. All of these can be adapted to an intensity appropriate to your fitness level. Kicks can be performed high or low; running can be geared to a low-impact level; and knee lifts can be done without jumping.

three walks or runs and a hop accented with a snap.

three walks or runs and a jump accented with a clap.

three walks or runs with a kick, with arms reaching either vertically or horizontally.

three walks or runs and a pivot.

Jump reach—jump followed by a hop with your leg extending to the side and your arms reaching diagonally away from your extended leg.

Hopscotch—a combination of a jump and a hop, with your lifted leg crossing behind your hopping leg. This movement alternates hopping feet.

Jump-kick—your kicking leg can kick to the front, side, or back. You can use a variety of arm patterns or perform claps under or over your leg.

Knee lift then jump-kick-jump.

Hop, touching your heel with your opposite hand, then jump-hop combined with a knee lift–jump.

AEROBIC ROUTINES AND MUSIC

Aerobic routines are the main challenge and excitement of the floor aerobic class because they enable participants to "dance their hearts out."

Most aerobic routines are performed with the leader at the front of the class and the group facing the leader, but variations of group formations add novelty to the daily workout regimens. Dances can be performed in a circle, with a partner, or in two lines facing each other (such as the Virginia reel). Group interaction can add much energy to the class and encourage a sense of classroom community. The instructor should not always be performing with the class; in addition

ACTIVE WARM-UP ROUTINE

Movement	Repetitions	Counts
March in place	8	1 each (total: 8)
3 walks and a hop	1 time forward and backward	4 each (total: 8)
Grapevine and a clap	4, alternating right and left	4 each (total: 8)
Jazz square	2	4 each (total: 8)
		Total: 32

WARM-UP AEROBIC ROUTINES

Steps	Repetitions	Counts
PATTERN 1		
1. Grapevine	right, left	4 each (total: 16)
2. Lunge sideways with arm punches	4, alternating right and left	2 each (total: 8)
3. Mambo	2	4 each (total: 8)
		Total: 32
PATTERN 2		
1. 3 runs and a jump-clap, forward and backward	1	(total: 8)
2. 3 step-turns and a clap	2, right and left	(total: 8)
3. Repeat 3 runs and a jump-clap, forward and backward	1	(total: 8)
4. Repeat 3 step-turns and a clap	2, right and left	(total: 8)
		Total: 32

to leading floor aerobic routines, it is the instructor's responsibility to correct posture and alignment, to assist students with the execution of steps, and to monitor, as much as possible, individual pace.

Aerobic routines are performed to specially arranged aerobic music that combines popular songs that have a steady beat and lively tempo. A *phrase* of aerobic movement is a combination of 4 sets of 8 counts, for a total of 32 beats of music.

PEAK AEROBIC ROUTINES

Steps	Repetitions	Counts
PATTERN 1		
1. Flea-hop	8	1 each (total: 8)
2. Breakaways	4, alternating right and left	2 each (total: 8)
3. 4 runs and 2 pivots	1	(total: 8)
4. Jump-kick	4, alternating legs	2 in combination (total: 8)
		Total: 32
PATTERN 2		
1. Side leap right and jump-clap	3 2	2 each (total: 6) 1 each (total: 2)
2. Side leap left and jump-clap	3 2	2 each (total: 6) 1 each (total: 2)
3. Pony	8, alternating right and left	2 each (total: 16)
		Total: 32

The choreography of a floor aerobic routine consists of several movement phrases repeated many times. A change in phrase in a floor aerobic routine is often determined by the music. The steps and movements are then choreographed in beats of 8: for example, jog 8 counts, jump 8 counts, hop and kick 8 counts, and so on.

Each phase of the aerobic workout requires a different tempo of music. **Tempo** is defined as the speed at which the music is played and is measured in beats per minute. In other words, the slower the tempo, or speed, of the song, the fewer beats per minute will occur. Count the beats of the music as you would your pulse.

The warm-up, stretch, low-impact, and cool-down routines require moderate or walking-paced music. This is measured at a range of 110 to 140 BPM (beats per minute). Peak aerobic routine tempos vary in range from 140 to 160 BPM. This is considered a jogging pace. Body toning and conditioning music should stay in a range of 110 to 130 BPM.

Premade aerobic tapes may be purchased through specialty aerobic catalogs. The music is easy to follow and continuous, and the beats per minute are usually listed. Oftentimes, for each song, the appropriate phase of the workout is included, for example, warm-up, aerobic warm-up, peak aerobics. For your own personal workouts, these tapes work well as they guide you through all the phases of a class at the appropriate tempos.

With your favorite music and combination of aerobic movements and steps, you can easily develop your own aerobic routines. Varying levels of aerobic routines are outlined. You can alter the choreography of these sample routines by adding or deleting repetitions of the movement phrases.

AEROBIC COOL-DOWN ROUTINES

Steps	Repetitions	Counts
PATTERN 1		
1. Lunges	2 right, 2 left	2 each (total: 8)
2. March	8	1 each (total: 8; *note* the last 2 counts have 3 steps with the rhythm 1 and 2 to change feet)
3. Lunges	2 left, 2 right	4 each (total: 8)
4. March	8	1 each (total: 8; *note* the last 2 counts have 3 steps with the rhythm 1 and 2 to change feet)
		Total: 32
PATTERN 2		
1. Slide forward, alternating right and left	4	2 each (total: 8)
2. Walk backward, with backward shoulder rolls	8	1 each (total: 8)
3. Slide forward, alternating right and left	4	2 each (total: 8)
4. Walk backward, with backward shoulder rolls	8	1 each (total: 8)
		Total: 32

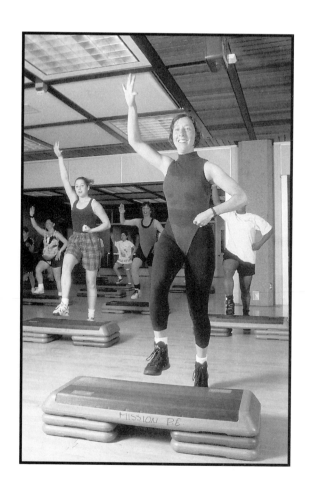

9

STEP AEROBICS

Step aerobics became popular in the late 1980s. Gin Miller, a retired gymnast, was using the step as a means for rehabilitation from injury. In the process of using the step, she began to realize its vast potential for fitness training choreography. Prior to this time, the step was mainly used as a testing tool for fitness evaluations such as the Step Test (fitness worksheet p. W-13). When Gin began to expand on the choreographic possibilities of the step as a means for fitness, her ideas caught on immediately with the fitness industry. Her introduction was the beginning of a craze that is still extremely popular today.

Step aerobics follows the same fitness rules as floor or dance aerobics. Instead of traveling on the floor, you use a bench or "step" to achieve the aerobic workout. In a step class, you perform a series of step routines or combinations in which you step up and down from the bench in time to upbeat, yet moderately paced music. The step can provide a low-impact, high-energy workout with added emphasis on the lower body, particularly the muscles of the hips, buttocks, and legs. In this chapter, we will describe the step class as well as the many movements used in the workout. Musical selection as well as variety on the step are also discussed.

THE STEP

The step equipment should be sturdy as well as slip- and skid-proof. Typically, your school or fitness center will provide the step. For personal use, many commercial brands are available through fitness supply stores, fitness catalogs, and even local athletic stores. Risers are placed under the step platform to increase the intensity of the workout. When you are using the risers, it is important that the platform of the step is firmly locked into place. The positions around the step are identified as front, back, side, or ends.

THE STEP CLASS

In a typical step class, set up your step in a place where you can see the instructor and there is space around all sides of the step. If using risers, always check that the platform is fully locked into place. The warm-up begins the class and may be done with or without the step. As in any aerobics class, it's important to warm up thoroughly before beginning the aerobic phase of the workout. In a step workout, the warm-up should concentrate specifically on the calves, quadriceps, hamstrings, buttocks muscles, and lower back. Ideally, in order to fulfill the principle of specificity, the warm-up will introduce some step moves. This may be the time when the instructor introduces new movements at half the speed. The step or bench can also double as a warm-up prop, which you can lean on for stretching. Once the warm-up is completed, the step workout begins. At this point in the class, you will perform the various step moves and patterns. Floor aero-bic movements can be interspersed in the step class to add variety and vary the intensity.

The aerobic cool-down follows the peak aerobic phase of the class. Just as you can use the step for warming up and stretching, it is also an excellent tool for cooling down. This is another opportunity for the instructor to review new movements at half time. It is also the time to use the step as a bench for body toning and deep stretching movements.

DETERMINING INTENSITY

The step class can accommodate students of any fitness level. Even a beginner can start the class just by using the platform without the risers. As your fitness level improves, you can increase the height of the bench or step. The number of risers used under the step platform determines the intensity of the workout. It is highly recommended that you use no more than two risers. Other ways to increase the intensity of the workout are by using the arms and adding propulsion or small jumps to the movements.

Individuals with knee problems should be very cautious on the step. The step workout may cause additional stress on knee and ankle joints. If you need to modify your workout,

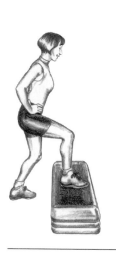
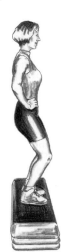
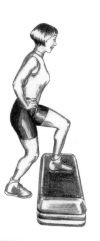
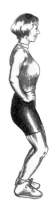

Basic step

whether for fitness level or injury prevention or care, lower the step so less flexion occurs at the knee and ankle joints.

TECHNIQUES FOR STEPPING

Certain step techniques are encouraged when performing the step workout:

- Make sure you place your whole foot on the step and step to the center of the platform.
- When stepping down, roll through the foot from ball of the foot to heel.
- Keep the step in your line of vision at all times.
- Slightly bend your knees at all times when stepping.
- Choose an appropriate step height; the knee should never flex beyond 90 degrees when stepping.
- Never step up or down with your back toward the step.
- At the conclusion of the step workout, use proper lifting techniques for returning the step to storage. When lifting the step, bend the knees and carry the step close to your body.

STEP MOVEMENTS

The step workout, like the aerobic workout, offers a wide variety of movement patterns.

BASIC STEP

Right foot up; left foot up; right foot down; left foot down.

When the same foot continues to lead a pattern repeatedly, that is called a *single foot lead*. When the lead foot alternates each time on the stepping up, that pattern is referred to as *alternating step*. To achieve an alternating step, a step variation called a tap must be used. To perform a *tap*, touch the floor (or step) with the ball of the foot and then immediately use that same foot to step up or down.

TAP DOWN

Right foot up; left foot up; right foot down; left foot down tap. Left foot up; right foot up; left foot down; right foot down tap.

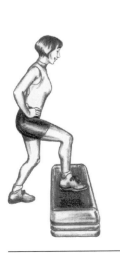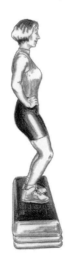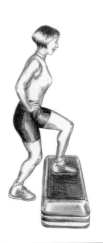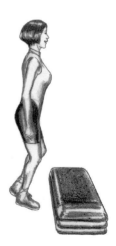

Tap down

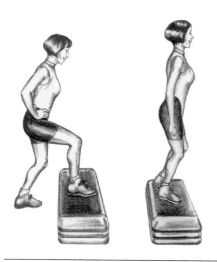

Tap up

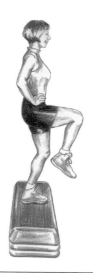

Knee up

TAP UP

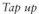

Right foot up; left foot up tap; left foot down; right foot down. Left foot up; right foot up tap; right foot down; left foot down.

Other step patterns or movements may be similarly created by changing the position of the leg lift.

KNEE UP

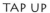

Right foot up; left knee lifts up; left foot down; right foot down. Left foot up; right knee up; right foot down; left foot down.

As you see, this pattern alternates the lead foot. Now you can perform this with the lifted leg kicking forward, lifting to the side, doing a leg curl to the rear, a straight leg lift to the rear, and so forth.

Variations on the leg lift also occur in repeater moves.

REPEATERS

Right foot up; left leg lift (any position); touch ball of left foot to floor; left leg lift; repeat left ball of foot to floor; left leg lift;

left foot down; right foot down. This is a repeater three, because the leg is lifted three times. Do not do more than five repeaters, because this can put too much stress on the knee and ankle joints. This movement can be performed either facing the front or on the diagonals.

Step patterns are also created either by widening the leg stance position, turning or rotating the body, facing a different direction, or traveling in different directions across or over the step. Following are some common step patterns that utilize these elements.

V STEP

Right foot up wide position; left foot up wide position; right foot down center; left foot down center.

TURN STEP OR $\frac{1}{2}$ TURN

Foot position is like the V step but with a turn of the body and a tap step; this pattern alternates lead foot: Right foot up wide; left foot up wide; right foot down at left corner, turning body to right; left foot down tap.

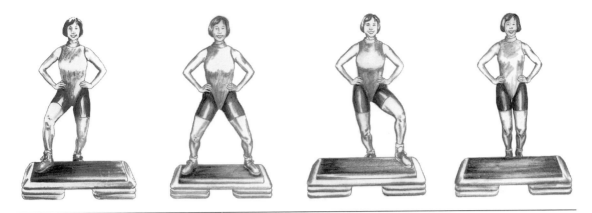

V step

Left foot up wide; right foot up wide; left foot down at right corner, turning body to left; right foot down tap.

L STEP

Begin this step off-center. Right foot up (off-center right); left foot up; right foot down to the right end of the box; left foot down tap. Left foot up (moving sideward); right foot up (moving sideward); left foot down; right foot down *tap*, to repeat the sequence on the same foot lead, or right foot *down*, to alternate to left foot lead. If alternating foot lead, continue: Left foot up (off-center left); right foot up; left foot down to the left end of the box; right foot down tap. Right foot up (moving sideward); left foot

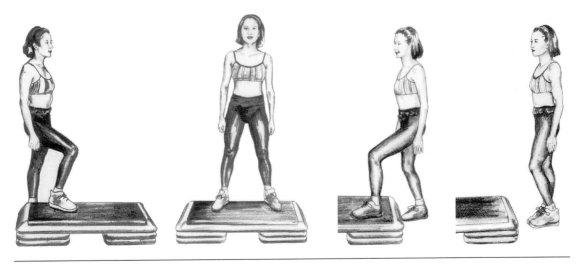

Turn step or $\frac{1}{2}$ turn

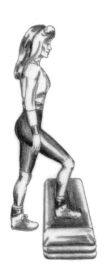
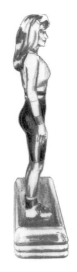
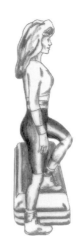
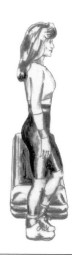

L step

up (moving sideward); right foot down; left foot down.

OVER THE TOP

Begin with the left side of the body parallel to the step. Left foot up; right foot up; left foot down on the back side of the step; right foot down tap. To return to the front of the step: Right foot up; left foot up; right foot down on the front side of the step; left foot down tap.

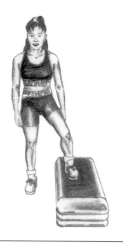
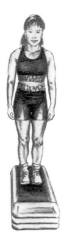
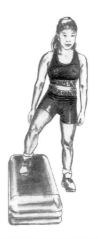
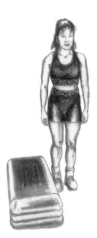

Over the top

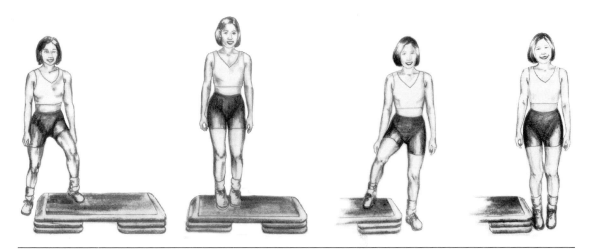

Across the top

ACROSS THE TOP

Begin at the left end of the box. Right foot up; left foot up; right foot down on the right end of the step; left foot down tap. To return to the left end of the step: Left foot up; right foot up; left foot down on the left end of the step; right foot down tap.

CORNER TO CORNER

This movement traverses across the diagonal of the step. Begin this step off-center, facing the diagonal. Step right foot up; step left to opposite corner of the step; step right foot down; step left foot down.

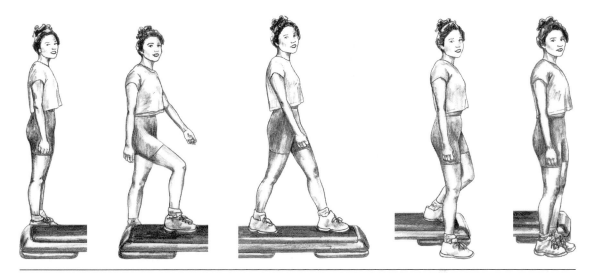

Corner to corner

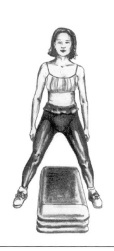
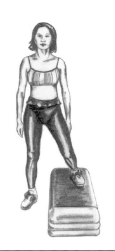
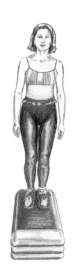

Straddle up

STRADDLE UP

Start from a position straddling the step: Right foot up; left foot up to end on top of the step.

STRADDLE DOWN

Start from a position standing sideways on the top of the step: Right foot down on the right side of the step; left foot down on the left side of the step.

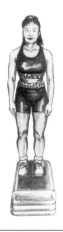
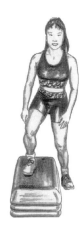
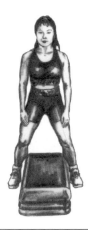

Straddle down

AROUND THE WORLD

This movement traverses around the whole step and is one of the more vigorous moves. Begin at the middle of the step, facing forward. Right foot up; left knee up with $\frac{1}{4}$ turn to the side of the step; left foot down; right foot tap; right foot up; left knee up with $\frac{1}{4}$ turn to the back of the step; left foot down; right foot down; right foot up; left knee up with $\frac{1}{4}$ turn to the other side of the step; left foot down; right foot tap; right foot up; left knee up with $\frac{1}{4}$ turn to the front of the step; left foot down; right foot tap. You have completed one pattern of Around the World.

T-STEP

Begin by facing the side of the step. Right foot up; left foot up; right foot straddle; left foot straddle; right foot up; left foot up; right foot down; left foot down. (This is a combination of the Basic and Straddle Steps.)

LUNGES

Lunges can be performed from any of the positions on the step. The lunge can be performed with one foot lunging onto the step and the opposite leg on the floor. A lunge can also be performed from the top of the step with a one foot lunge off the step to the floor. When performing the lunge off the step, make sure that only the ball of the foot touches the floor, keeping the heel slightly off the floor.

SQUATS

Squats can be performed on top of the step in a wide stance. Squats can also be performed with one foot on the step and the other foot on the floor. This is called the *split squat*.

Both the lunge and the squat can be used in step routines as well as with the step during body toning.

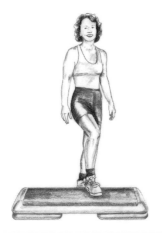

Step onto the platform

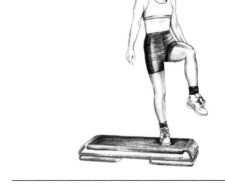

Knee lift with $\frac{1}{4}$ turn to corner

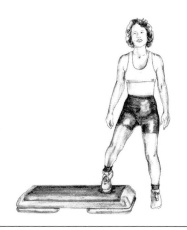

Step off the platform

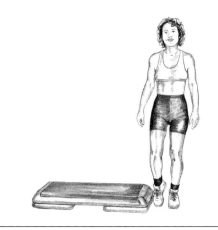

Tap down

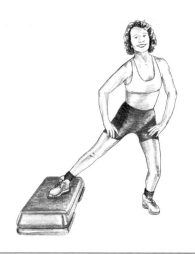

Lunges

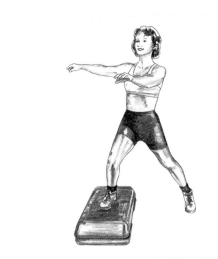

CREATING VARIETY WITH STEP MOVEMENTS

You can vary step patterns by altering the direction in which the body faces the step. You can use step movements *from the front, from the* *side, from the end, from the corner, from astride,* or *from the top.* You can also create step pattern variations by combining some of the basic step patterns outlined above. You can also vary the step by incorporating step work

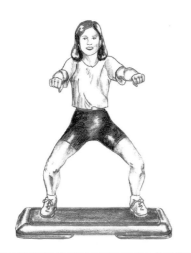

Squat—"on box"

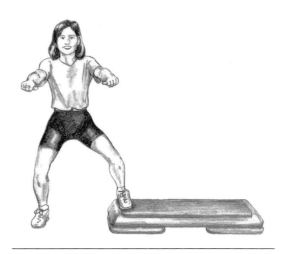

Squat—"off box"

with aerobic movements done in an aerobics class, thus doing some patterns on the step and some patterns on the floor. All steps can be made more difficult by adding a variety of arm movement exercises and patterns. All steps become more intense when propulsion is added to the step. *Propulsion* occurs when both feet push off the ground or off the step, exchanging positions during the airborne phase of the movement. Because propulsion steps are high-impact movements, it is *not* advisable to use propulsion steps as a beginning step aerobicizer or to use propulsion steps with weights.

As outlined, each step routine is 32 counts. When the instructor first teaches the routine, each step may be repeated many times until the students feel comfortable with the movement. Once all the steps have been mastered, then they may be condensed to the 32-count phrase in order to experience the fun and variety in the choreography.

MUSICAL SELECTION

The step aerobic class requires a much slower tempo than the floor aerobic class. The ideal BPM (beats per minute) for a step class should be between 122–127 BPM. Some teachers like to go faster (up to 135 BPM), but research has shown that this can be dangerous. Rather than increasing the musical BPM, you can raise intensity by adding risers to the platform, moving around the step, using propulsion moves, and/or increasing the use and level of the arms. Just as for floor aerobics, ready-made tapes are available for the step class. Catalogs are available from companies that sell these ready-made tapes (see Appendix D).

The step workout appeals to both men and women; it is a continuous challenge both

STEP ROUTINES

Steps	Repetitions	Counts
ROUTINE ONE		
1. Basic step	2 right, 2 left	4 each (total: 16)
2. V step	1 right, 1 left	4 each (total: 8)
3. Basic step	1 right	4 total
4. Knee up	1 right	4 total
Repeat, starting with basic step left.		
ROUTINE TWO		
1. L step	1 right, 1 left	8 each (total: 16)
2. Repeater with side leg	1 right	8 total
3. Kick leg front	1 left, 1 right	4 each (total: 8)
Repeat, starting with L step left.		
ROUTINE THREE		
1. Half-turn or turn step	right, left, right, left	4 each (total: 16)
2. Over the top	1 right, 1 left, 1 right	4 each (total: 12)
3. Tap up, tap down	1 left	4 total
Repeat all, starting at the back of the step with the left foot.		
ROUTINE FOUR		
1. T step	2 with right leading	8 each (total: 16)
2. Knee up	Right, left, right	4 each (total: 12)
3. Basic step	left	4 total
Repeat, starting with T step on the left.		

mentally and physically. It adds variety to fitness programs, provides a total body workout, and is vigorous enough for a maximum challenge.

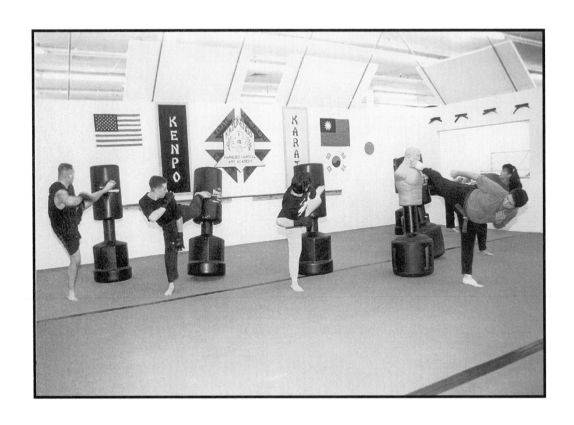

10

BODY TONING AND CONDITIONING

The body toning and conditioning phase of the class promotes muscular strength and endurance. During this phase, equal time must be devoted to all the body's muscle groups (Figure 10-1). Body toning exercises improve the initial tone of the muscles as well as their endurance capabilities. Conditioning exercises place increased demand on muscle fibers in order to improve actual muscular strength. This session of the class is approximately 15 to 20 minutes long; the time may vary, depending on the individual instructor's format. Exercises to work specific areas of the body (arms, waist, abdomen, legs, and buttocks) should be blended into the workout with smooth transitions to make the body toning and conditioning phase

more enjoyable. The format emphasizes exercises for one body area at a time.

When referring to body toning, we are actually referring to muscle toning. *Muscle tone* is the natural tension within a muscle, even when the muscle is relaxed. Muscular contraction, the tightening or shortening of a muscle, will contour and tone muscles. Muscles that are not used regularly will atrophy and look loose and flabby.

Body toning exercises do not burn body fat; only aerobic exercise burns fat. Exercises that contract and strengthen the muscles give the figure shape and form.

Strengthening and toning exercises are those that are performed against a force or resistance;

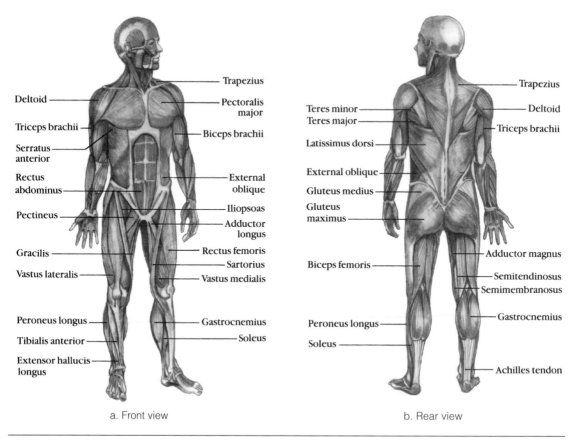

FIGURE 10-1   *The body's muscle groups*

that resistance may be in the form of pushing, pulling, or lifting your own body part or a weight.

It is important to note that even when you are performing an exercise for a specific muscle, other muscles are also involved. The muscle that is the prime mover of the exercise is termed the **agonist.** The opposing muscle group that is usually stretched while the prime mover is contracted is termed the **antagonist.** Muscle groups that assist but are not the prime movers in an exercise are termed **synergists.** It is important to make each muscle an agonist and antagonist during your workout, so that muscular balance is achieved.

STRENGTH OR ENDURANCE?

Body toning exercises can improve both muscular endurance and muscular strength. Outlined in Chapter 4 were training principles used as a means to improve fitness. These fitness principles must be applied when you are performing toning exercises. If your goal is to develop muscular strength, then you must perform each exercise with heavy resistance but execute only a few repetitions of the exercise. If your goal is to develop muscular endurance, use a light resistance and perform many repetitions of the exercise.

STRENGTH——————ENDURANCE

Heavy resistance, few repetitions	Light-moderate resistance, many repetitions

Strength gains occur when you work at 50 to 100 percent of your *maximum repetition* (abbreviated *1 RM*), or how much weight you can lift in one all-out exertion. If you are working to build strength, ideally you should perform 1–5 sets of an exercise at 50 to 100 percent of 1 RM, and you should do 3–8 repetitions of each set. Endurance, on the other hand, will improve if you do 1–5 sets of the exercise at 20 to 70 percent of your 1 RM, and 8–25 repetitions of each set.

For muscle toning, we generally work in the middle of the continuum drawn above, performing 1–3 sets of the exercises at about 40 to 70 percent of your 1 RM and 8–15 repetitions for each set performed. When working in this manner, you should choose a resistance that makes the last few repetitions difficult to perform. When all the repetitions are easy, it is time to apply overload either by adding another set or increasing the resistance.

TYPES OF MUSCLE CONTRACTIONS

In the typical aerobics class, two types of muscle contractions are used. Both are effective for developing strength and endurance. Both also have their disadvantages as well as advantages.

Isometric Contraction

An **isometric contraction** is a muscular contraction where tension is created in the muscle but there is no movement. You are actually holding the weight in a specific position. The weight you are holding may be your own body weight, hand-held weights, or a type of resistance equip-

ment. For strength to be increased with an isometric contraction, you must use a heavy resistance, maintaining the contracted position for 6–8 seconds. For endurance to be increased, maintain the contraction for 10–20 seconds, using a light weight or no weight at all. *People with high blood pressure should not perform isometric contractions, because they do stop the blood flow.*

One disadvantage to isometric contraction is that it develops the strength and endurance only at the specific angle you are holding. To improve fitness levels at the other joint positions, you would have to repeat the contraction at all the angles of the joint. To develop strength and endurance through the complete range of motion, you should perform the exercises doing isotonic contractions.

Isotonic Contraction

An **isotonic contraction** develops tension in the muscle as the muscle moves through its complete range of motion. This type of contraction has two phases, concentric and eccentric. A **concentric contraction** involves a shortening of the joint angle. An **eccentric contraction** involves increasing the angle of the joint. For example, in the hamstring curl, bending the leg and bringing the heel toward the buttocks is the concentric contraction of the exercise; straightening of the leg is the eccentric contraction.

To add overload to isotonic contractions, you can

1. Increase the weight or resistance
2. Perform the exercise at a slower pace
3. Increase the range of motion of the exercise

As an example, the curl-up is more difficult to do slowly. You can also make the curl-up more difficult by increasing the range of motion, that is, lifting the shoulders and upper back higher off the ground.

TYPES OF RESISTANCE

Resistance can be increased by using a more difficult body position, holding the position, going at a slower pace, adding light weights, using resistance tubing, or using weight machines. Typically, in the aerobics class, you would increase the resistance in any of these ways except with weight machines.

Free or Hand-Held Weights

Hand-held or ankle weights are a common form of resistance used in aerobics classes. They are easy to store and provide a fixed resistance; that is, the weight resistance remains the same throughout the entire range of motion of the exercise, so that when you lift a 3-pound weight, at all angles it will be 3 pounds. Free weights vary in their size or weight, thus allowing for a variety of resistance levels for exercisers. It is usually best to start with 1-pound hand-held weights and gradually progress to the 3-, 5-, and 10-pound weights. Light weights will build endurance. When working with light weights, either hand-held or ankle weights, follow these rules for a safe and effective workout:

1. Never swing the weights.

2. Do not squeeze the weights. Hold them firmly but gently. Holding the weights too tightly could be detrimental to your circulation.

3. Perform the exercises *slowly!* Control and tension are very important for building strength. Just going through the motions does not do the job; *tension* must be created in the muscle in order to build strength.

4. Work until the muscle is fatigued, but stop before it is in pain.

5. Perform exercises for the large muscle groups (for example, the deltoids and pectorals) before exercising the smaller muscle groups (for example, the biceps and triceps).

6. Perform 8 to 16 repetitions of an exercise before going on to a new exercise. Do a series of 3 or 4 different exercises for different muscle groups and then come back and repeat the series 2 or 3 more times.

7. Work the muscle group as well as its opposing muscle group (for example, hamstring and then quadricep or bicep and then tricep).

8. Allow a 1-minute rest of one muscle group before doing another exercise for that same group. For example, if you do an exercise for the biceps, do one next for the triceps before going back to a bicep exercise. Muscles need a rest after reaching fatigue.

9. Never hold your breath when performing any of the exercises. Breathe easily and naturally with each movement.

10. Remember to start with light weights, and always perform with proper technique.

Resistance Bands

Resistance bands are another effective way to increase strength and muscle endurance. With a band, unlike free weights, as you stretch it, the resistance increases. This type of resistance is called *variable resistance*. There are many types and brand names of exercise bands. The bands may be surgical tubing, heavy-duty office rubber bands, or wide sheets of rubber that resemble strips of an inner tube. Brand-name resistance bands come in different colors that represent the amount of resistance: either light, medium, or heavy. The office rubber bands come in different thicknesses; the thickness determines the intensity.

When working with resistance bands, there are certain techniques you should follow:

1. Always control the movement so that tension is created in the muscle and you are not working with momentum.

2. Maintain correct body alignment.

3. Never bend back the wrist when holding the band. Keep it in a straight position from the elbow.
4. Never let the band fly away. Keep it under control.
5. If you cannot perform at least 6 repetitions of a specific exercise, then lower the intensity of the resistance.
6. Increase the intensity of the band only when you can easily perform 10–15 repetitions of an exercise.

Body Positions

There are many ways you can use body position to increase the resistance of an exercise. When performing a push-up, the easiest version is done on the hands and knees (modified). To make this exercise progressively more difficult, perform it on your hands and with only your toes on the floor (standard), move the hands closer together on the floor or wider than the shoulders (this isolates specific muscles), or in the step workout, try doing it with the feet up on the step.

Leg lifts are another exercise in which position affects the difficulty. When performing leg-lift exercises lying on your side, the exercise is more difficult when the leg is straight than when the leg is bent.

Abdominal exercises, specifically curl-ups, are easiest with the arms at the side. As you bring the arms farther away from the body (behind or over the head), the exercise gets harder.

In the step workout, the use of the step is consistently a good means of altering the intensity level and resistance of an exercise.

EXERCISE EVALUATION

As you progress through the body toning and conditioning exercises introduced in this chapter, you may want to refer to Figure 9-1 to review which muscle group you are using and where it is located. In addition, it is important to evaluate each exercise you perform to gain the maximum benefits of that exercise. The exercises in this book have been evaluated for general safety, but since each one of us is unique, it is important that each exercise work specifically for you. To evaluate each exercise, answer the following five questions:

1. What is the purpose of this exercise?
2. How effective is this exercise in meeting that purpose?
3. Are there risks involved in performing this exercise?
4. Can I perform this exercise with proper technique?
5. Do I need to modify this exercise?

To complement the strengthening exercises, flexibility exercises should be included in the body toning and conditioning phase of the workout. These exercises should complement the toning and conditioning exercises by stretching previously exercised muscles. For maximum flexibility, the muscles must be stretched and worked through a full range of motion. Stretching exercises may include any of those described in Chapter 11. The combination of strengthening and stretching exercises is the ideal format for improving muscle tone and aesthetic appearance.

BODY TONING AND CONDITIONING EXERCISES

Arms and Shoulders

BICEPS CURL

major muscles used: **biceps brachii**

Stand in proper alignment, with your feet shoulder width apart and your knees slightly bent. Begin with your arms in an extended position at your sides, with your hands fisted. Bend your arms at the elbows until your hands come near your shoulders. Keep your elbows in contact with your waist. Return to the starting position.

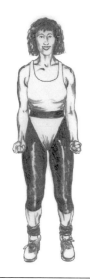
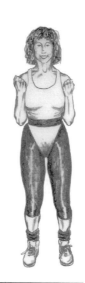

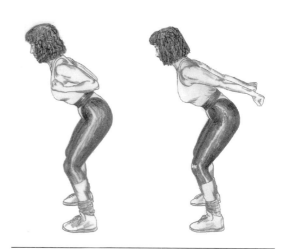

Biceps curl

Triceps kickback

PRECAUTIONS

- *Keep your upper arms and elbows close to your sides.*
- *Move your lower arms only.*

TRICEPS KICKBACK

major muscles used: **triceps brachii**
posterior aspect of the deltoid

Bend over at your waist until your upper torso is diagonal to the floor, with your feet shoulder width apart and your knees slightly bent. Keep your upper arms and elbows close to your sides. With your fisted palms facing each other, bend your lower arms up at a 45-degree angle to the upper arms. Then extend both arms behind your back until your elbows are straight. Return to the starting position.

PRECAUTIONS

- *Bend your knees so there is no pressure on the back. If back pain occurs, stop the exercise.*
- *Keep your body stationary and move only your lower arms.*

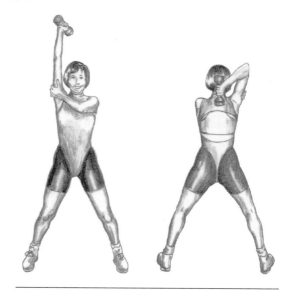

Triceps extension

TRICEPS EXTENSION

major muscles used: **triceps brachii**

Start in the same position as the biceps curl, but bring one hand over head. Bend that arm at the elbow so the hand almost touches between the shoulder blades. Support the arm with the opposite hand. Hold the arm near the tricep, either in front of the chest or behind the head. Extend the working arm that is bent to a straight position over head. Return to the starting position. Repeat with the other arm.

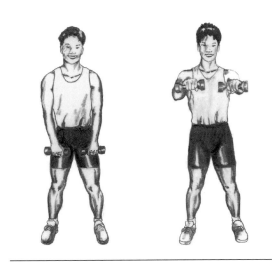

Forward arm raise

PRECAUTIONS

- *Have the arm you are working right by your ear.*
- *Maintain neutral alignment and bend the knees.*

FORWARD ARM RAISE

major muscle used: **anterior aspect of the deltoid**

Start in the same position as the biceps curl, but hold your arms in front of your thighs, fists facing inward. Lift your arms forward until they reach shoulder height, then return them to the starting position.

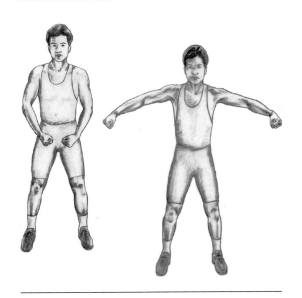

Side lateral raise

PRECAUTIONS

- *Do not lift arms higher than shoulder level.*
- *Avoid creating tension in the shoulders.*
- *Maintain neutral spine alignment.*

SIDE LATERAL RAISE

major muscle used: **middle aspect of the deltoid**

Start in the same position as the biceps curl, but hold your arms at your sides with your fists facing inward and your elbows slightly bent. Lift your arms out to the sides until they reach shoulder height, then return to the starting position.

PRECAUTION

Do not lift your arms above shoulder height as this may injure the shoulders.

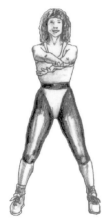

Palms down

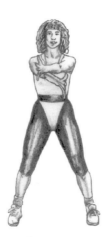

Palms side

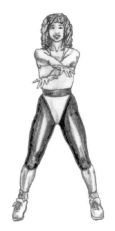

Palms up

Arm scissors

ARM SCISSORS

major muscles used: **anterior aspect of the
deltoid
pectoralis major**

In a standing position with your feet shoulder width apart, extend your arms forward from your chest and at shoulder height, with your palms down. "Scissor" your arms by alternately crossing one arm over the other. To exercise all muscles of the arms, vary the position of your palms: palms up, palms in, palms out.

═══ PRECAUTIONS ═══

- *Try not to elevate or tense the shoulders.*
- *Maintain correct alignment.*
- *Bend the knees slightly.*

UPRIGHT ROW

major muscles used: **middle aspect of the
deltoid
upper trapezius
biceps brachii**

Stand in proper alignment, with your feet shoulder width apart and your knees

slightly bent. Extend your arms downward in front of your body with your hands fisted or grasping weights about a hand's width apart and facing your body. Pull your hands up your chest until they reach your chin, your elbows extending out away from your body and, at the top of the movement, in an upward position. Slowly return to the starting position.

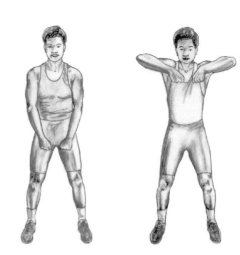

Upright row

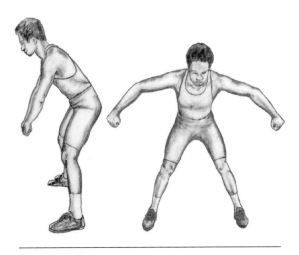

Upper back fly

UPPER BACK FLY

major muscles used: **middle trapezius
rhomboids**

Start in a wide, parallel stance, leaning forward, with your torso diagonal to the floor and your knees bent. Keep your focus toward the floor. Your arms should be straight or slightly bent, hanging from the shoulders, with your hands fisted. Open your arms to the sides and then return them to the starting position. Repeat several times, slowly and with resistance.

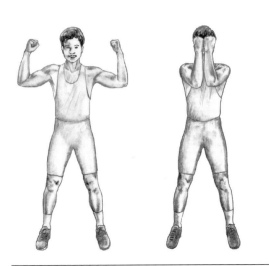

Pectoral press

Chest and Back

PECTORAL PRESS

major muscle used: **pectoralis major**

Stand with your feet shoulder width apart and your knees slightly bent. Bring your arms out to your sides below shoulder height and bend your elbows, with your forearms pointing upward and your hands fisted inward. Bring your arms together in front of your body until your elbows touch. Return slowly to the starting position.

MODIFIED PUSH-UP

major muscles used: **triceps brachii
pectoralis major**

Lie prone on the floor. Place your hands under your shoulders, with your fingers facing forward. Keep your feet together, legs bent at your knees. Keep your body in a straight plane from your knees to your head as you push your upper body off the floor until both your arms are completely straight. Lower your body back to the floor,

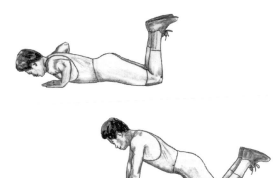

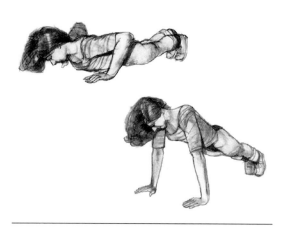

Modified push-up

Standard push-up

maintaining a straight plane. Repeat the modified push-up several times. See precautions following the standard push-up.

STANDARD PUSH-UP

major muscles used: **triceps brachii
pectoralis major**

Lie prone on the floor. Place your hands under your shoulders, with your fingers facing forward. Keep your feet together and flexed, with your body weight on the balls of your feet. Keep your body straight, abdominals and hip muscles contracted, as you push up until both your arms are straight. Lower your body halfway to the floor by bending your elbows, keeping your weight equally distributed on your hands and the balls of your feet. Repeat the push-up several times. In the step workout, place the balls of the feet on the step to increase exercise intensity.

PRECAUTIONS

- *To prevent placing undue strain on the vertebrae of your lower back, do not let your lower back arch.*
- *Do not raise your buttocks to dip your chin.*
- *Do not allow your hips to sag.*
- *Avoid locking your elbows at the top of the exercise.*
- *If this exercise is too difficult, just lower your body a few inches. Do not attempt to go all the way unless you can perform the push-up correctly. Gradually build up your strength.*

HORIZONTAL FLY AND PRESS

major muscle used: **pectoralis major**

Lie on your back with your knees bent and the soles of your feet on the floor. For the flys, extend the arms out to the side and very slowly bring them in front of your face. The palms will be facing. It is an arcing motion and the elbows are slightly bent.

For the press, your body is in the same position but the arms are bent with the

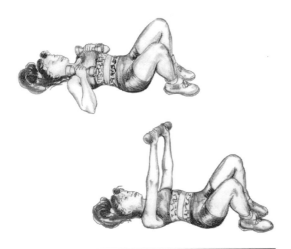

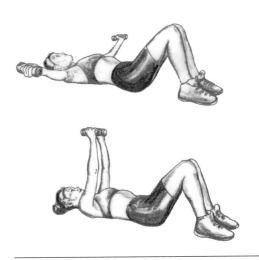

Horizontal press

Horizontal fly

hands by the side of the chest. From this position, press the arms straight out in front so they end with thumbs together in front of your face. Return to the starting position for both exercises and repeat.

You can combine the two exercises. When the thumbs are together at the end of the press, open the arms to the side for the start of the fly. Now perform the arcing motion of the fly and from here, bend the arms to the starting position of the press.

MOVEMENT TIPS

- *Perform these exercises from a step, so that the arms have farther to open on the fly and the elbows can bend open more on the press.*
- *By changing the angle of the step, you can perform incline and/or decline presses or flys.*

PULLOVERS

major muscles used: **pectoralis major**
latissimus dorsi
triceps brachii

Perform this exercise only when lying flat or on the incline step. Lie on your back with your knees bent and soles of your feet on the step. Extend your arms vertically at a level below the chest with the palms facing the ceiling and the elbows slightly bent. Slowly pull the arms over the head until they touch the floor. Return the arms to the starting position. The back will slightly arch in the pullover position. Make sure to press your back toward the step as you return to the starting position.

ONE-ARM BENT ROW

major muscles used: **latissimus dorsi**
posterior aspect of the deltoid
biceps brachii

Start in a lunge position with the body weight forward over the front leg and the support hand on the front thigh. Lean over with the hand-held weight and reach diagonally toward the floor. Pull that arm back with the elbow bent. The elbow should go behind the body, yet stay very close to the body (almost touching the body). Return slowly to the starting position. Repeat the exercise on the other side. In the step

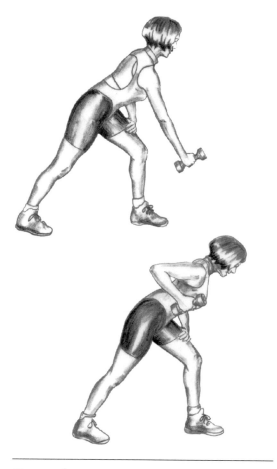

One-arm bent row

workout, perform this exercise with the front foot on the step.

PRECAUTIONS

- *Make sure the other hand rests on the thigh so that the back is supported.*
- *Make sure to pull the elbow as far back as possible.*
- *Maintain neutral neck alignment.*

SEATED ROW

major muscles used: **latissimus dorsi**
　　　　　　　　　　posterior aspect of the deltoid
　　　　　　　　　　biceps brachii

Sit on the floor with your legs crossed. With weights or other resistance in your hands, reach forward with both arms. Keeping the elbows close to your body, pull your hands to your waist. Repeat. In the step workout, perform this exercise while seated on the step.

PRECAUTIONS

- *Do not elevate the shoulders.*
- *Keep the elbows right at the side when you pull the arms in.*
- *Make sure to lean all the way forward to stretch the muscles you are working.*

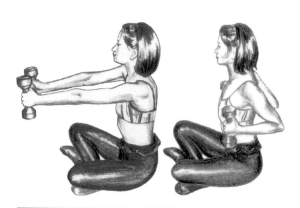

Seated row

Abdominals

The main muscle of the abdominal region is the long sheath called the *rectus abdominus*. This muscle attaches at the ribs at one end and the pubic bone at the other end. Whenever this muscle contracts, which happens when we flex or bend our spine, the entire muscle shortens. There are exercises that emphasize more stress on the upper third or lower third of the muscle, although the entire muscle contracts. If you hear someone say, "this exercise works our lower abdominals," understand that there are no lower or upper abdominals but that the exercise is merely putting emphasis on the lower region.

The other muscles of the abdominal area are the *internal* and *external oblique abdominals*. This group runs across the rib cage and attaches to the edges of the pubic bone. There is one on each side of the body. The function of the obliques is to rotate the spine. Whenever we do twisting movements, these muscles are activated.

The last set of abdominal muscles is a deep muscle that lies under the rectus abdominus and the obliques. This muscle, called the *transverse abdominal*, is used mainly for posture. When you maintain good alignment as discussed in Chapter 5, this muscle group maintains its tone.

In order to strengthen and tone the rectus abdominus, the spine must be flexed. In full sit-ups, where the entire spine is lifted off the floor, you are actually strengthening the muscles that flex the hip on the last half of the exercise. It is only the initial lift that contracts the rectus abdominus. Curl-ups or half sit-ups are the appropriate exercises for the rectus abdominus. Variations on this exercise make it more fun, but the actual action is still the same, trunk flexion.

To concentrate on the obliques, you perform an exercise that twists or rotates the trunk as you lift the torso from the ground. Again, variations are merely a way to make the work more fun and sometimes more difficult.

For all abdominal exercises, apply overload by

1. Changing the arm positions (farther from the body is harder)
2. Lifting the torso higher from the ground
3. Performing each exercise at a slower pace
4. Performing the exercises on a decline step

As with all toning exercises, it is important to maintain tension in the abdominals at all times to receive maximum benefits from the exercise.

CURL-UP

Lie on your back, clasp your hands behind your head, and keep your elbows back. Bend your knees, placing the soles of your

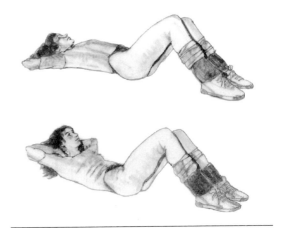

Curl-up

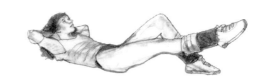

One-leg-straight curl-up

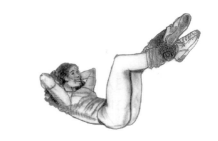

Two-leg curl-up

feet firmly on the floor. Take a deep breath. Exhale and then contract your abdominals and press your lower back to the floor as you sit up halfway, lifting your head and shoulders off the floor. Lower shoulders to the ground only before repeating the exercise.

Variations
Hands reach to knees
Hands crossed at the chest

One leg to the ceiling

Both legs to the ceiling and crossed at the ankles

Legs to the ceiling and slightly spread apart

ABDOMINAL CURL-DOWN

Begin in a sitting position, with your knees bent and your feet flat on the floor. Relax your arms at the sides of your body. Slowly lower your torso to the floor by rounding your back, contracting your stomach muscles, and placing one vertebra at a time on the floor. The end position is with only the head off the ground. At this point you roll back up to the starting position. Make sure the chin stays close to the chest at all times.

DOUBLE CURL

Lie on your back, bend your legs, clasp your hands behind your head, and keep your elbows back. Lift your bent legs off the floor, and then lift your head and shoulders off the floor until your elbows touch your knees. Release your torso slightly away from your knees, but do *not* return to the floor. When you lift your knees you must also lift your hips off the ground. Do not use momentum to lift the hips.

PRECAUTION

Do not let your lower back arch off the floor.

OBLIQUE CURL

Start in the same position as the curl-up, but place one arm behind your head for support and reach the other arm out to the side on the floor. Lift the elbow and chest, and cross it to touch the opposite knee. Lower until only the head is off the ground and then repeat. Repeat on the other side.

Variations

One leg to ceiling; opposite hand touches toes of opposite foot

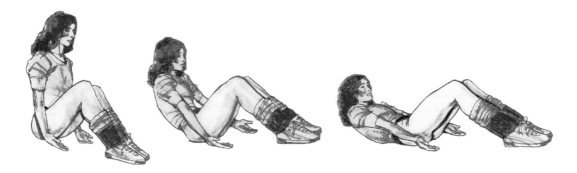

Abdominal curl-down

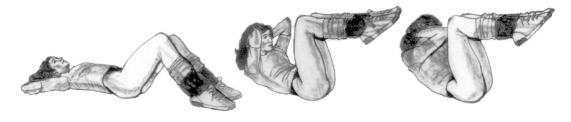

Double curl

Both knees to chest and both hands behind head; touch opposite elbow to opposite knee in a bicycle motion

Legs to ceiling and crossed at ankles, hands behind head; touch opposite elbow to opposite knee

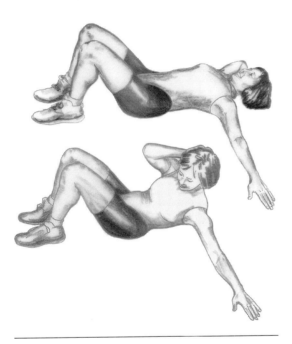

Oblique curl

SIDE BENDS

Start in the same position as for the curl-up, but with hands at the side on the floor. Reach as far to the right ankle with the right hand as possible. Repeat with the left side. The head is lifted off the floor for the entire exercise. The hands stay close to the ground.

Lower Body

STARTING POSITION FOR ALL LEG LIFTS

On your hands and knees, lift one leg so that it extends straight behind you, at hip level. Lower your head by bending your elbows and leaning forward, placing your body weight over your forearms.

STRAIGHT-LEG LIFT

major muscle used: **gluteus maximus**

From the starting position, lift your leg up several inches, and then lower it to hip level. Repeat exercise with your other leg.

BENT-LEG LIFT AND EXTENSION

major muscle used: **gluteus maximus**

From the starting position, bring the knee of your extended leg into your chest, and then extend your leg behind you, returning

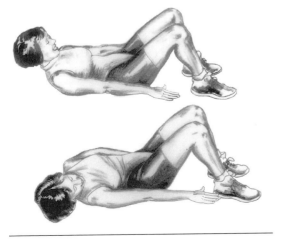

Side bends

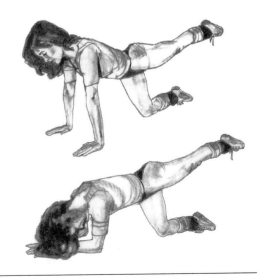

Starting position for leg-lift exercises

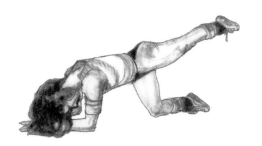

Straight-leg lift

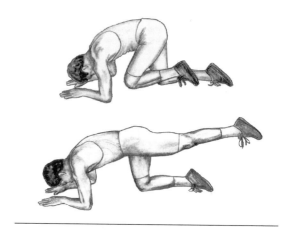

Bent-leg lift and extension

your leg to hip level. Repeat the exercise with your other leg.

BENT-KNEE LEG LIFT

major muscles used: **hamstrings
gluteus maximus**

From the starting position, bend the knee of your lifted leg with your foot flexed (the sole of your foot faces the ceiling). Lift your leg in this position several inches; then lower it to hip level. Repeat with your other leg.

PRECAUTIONS

- *Keep your back straight by contracting your abdominal muscles to avoid placing stress or strain on your lower back.*
- *Do not lift your leg above hip level when you are on your hands and knees. By lowering your head and shifting your body weight to your forearms, you can raise your leg without tilting your pelvis or placing stress on the lumbar disk.*
- *Keep your hips level. Avoid turning the working hip out.*

MOVEMENT TIP

All of the leg-lift exercises can be performed in a standing position, facing a wall or a ballet barre.

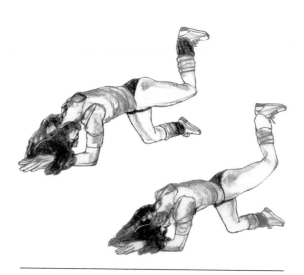

Bent-knee leg lift

CROSSOVER

major muscles used: **hip abductors (gluteus
medius and minimus)**

Lie on your right side, your body lying flat on the floor, with your right arm extended over your head. Bend your right knee so that your thigh is in line with your torso. Raise your left leg up with your foot flexed; then lower your leg at a comfortable angle in front of you to 3 inches above the floor. Continue to lift and lower your leg in this position with your leg slightly forward.

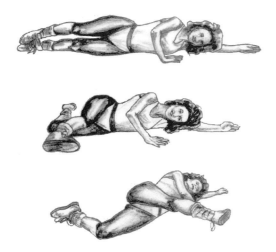

Crossover

Keep your hips square (not rolling forward or backward) throughout the exercise. Turn to your opposite side and repeat the crossover.

SIDE THIGH LIFT

major muscles used: **hip abductors (gluteus medius and minimus)**

Lie on your right side, with your right arm extended flat along the floor. Bend your right knee so that your knee and thigh remain in line with your torso. Keeping your left leg straight with your foot flexed, toes and knee facing forward, lift your leg 1 to 2 feet off the floor. (By keeping your knee and foot facing forward, you cannot lift your leg very high. Avoid turning your knee and foot up toward the ceiling.) Continue to lift and lower your leg in this posi-

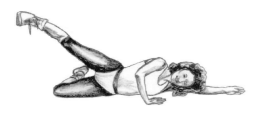

Side thigh lift

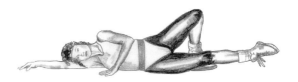

Inner thigh lift

tion. Turn to your opposite side and repeat the side thigh lift.

INNER THIGH LIFT

major muscles used: **hip abductors (brevis, longus, and magnus)**

Lie on your right side, with your right arm extended flat along the floor. Bend your left knee, and place your left foot flat on the floor behind your right knee. Keeping your right leg straight with your foot flexed, toes and knee facing forward, lift your right leg as high as possible. Repeat the exercise several times. Turn to your opposite side and repeat the inner thigh lift.

INNER THIGH BUTTERFLY

major muscles used: **hip abductors gluteus maximus**

Lie on your back with your knees bent, your feet apart, the soles of your feet firmly

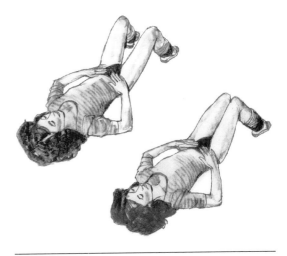

Inner thigh butterfly

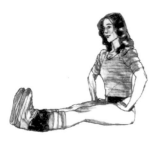
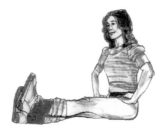

Front thigh lift

on the floor, and your hips lifted slightly off the floor. Close your knees, pressing your inner thighs together. Separate your knees approximately 12 inches. Do not let the soles of your feet lift off the floor. Repeat the close-open motion several times.

> **PRECAUTIONS**
> - *Do not let your lower back lift off the floor.*
> - *Do not hold your breath.*

FRONT THIGH LIFT

major muscles used: **quadriceps**

Start in a sitting position, with your legs straight forward and your feet flexed. Lift one leg slightly off the floor (2 to 3 inches). From this position, lift your leg up and down in a pulsing motion several times. Reverse the front thigh lift to your opposite leg.

> **PRECAUTIONS**
> - *Keep your back erect.*
> - *Do not lock your knees.*

PLIÉ

major muscles used: **hip abductors**
                               gluteus maximus
                               quadriceps

Start with your feet shoulder width apart and turned out from the hip joints about 45

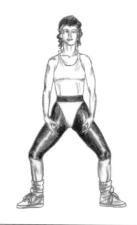

Plié

to 60 degrees. Keep your heels on the ground and your back and neck erect. Bend your knees as low as you can in this position. Return to the starting position by squeezing the inner thighs together. This exercise is taken from ballet and can be done in conjunction with upper body exercises.

> **PRECAUTIONS**
> - *Do not bend at your waist.*
> - *Make sure your knees go out over your toes.*
> - *Do not allow your buttocks to protrude. Keep them in line with your spine and maintain your pelvis in a neutral position.*

SQUAT

major muscles used: **quadriceps**
hamstrings
gluteus maximus

Start with your feet about shoulder width apart and in a parallel position. You can place your hands on your shoulders. Pitch your head and torso forward as if you were going to sit in a chair. Keep your head up and your back in a straight line as you lower your buttocks until your thighs are parallel to the floor. Pause and then return to the starting position.

PRECAUTIONS

- *Do not round your back during this exercise. Keep it elongated.*
- *Keep your knees in line with your toes.*

MOVEMENT TIP

When performing the squat, simultaneously do one of the upper-body exercises described. For example, you can perform a squat as you do an upright row or pectoral press. This saves time and works two groups of muscles at once.

LUNGE

major muscles used: **quadriceps**
hamstrings
gluteus maximus

Begin with your feet shoulder width apart and your hands resting on your shoulders. Lunge forward on your right foot until your thigh is almost parallel to the floor, your left knee still in line with your left ankle. Return to the starting position, using the buttocks muscles to push off the floor. Repeat 8 to 16 repetitions on one leg before repeating on the other side, or alternate every time.

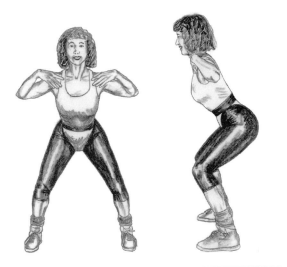

Squat

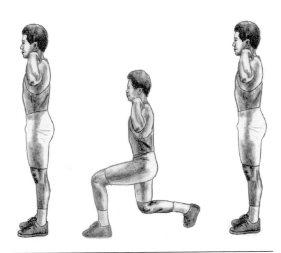

Lunge

MOVEMENT TIP

In the step workout, increase the intensity of the lunge by using the step.
Variations of the lunge using the step include

- *forward lunge onto the step*
- *sideward lunge onto the step*
- *stationary lunge with the back leg on the step*

HEEL RAISES

major muscle used: **gastrocnemius**

Stand with your feet in a parallel position about shoulder width apart. Rise onto the balls of your feet as far as possible, and then slowly lower to the starting position. Keep the knees as straight as possible. Hold on to a bar or wall for support if balance is a problem.

BENT-KNEE HEEL RAISES

major muscle used: **soleus (deep muscle of the calf)**

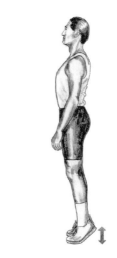

Heel raise

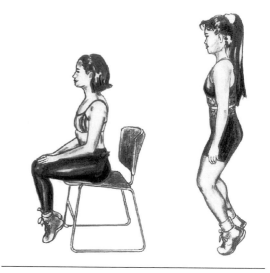

Bent-knee heel raise

This exercise can be done from a chair or in a standing position. If sitting, keep the spine neutral with the feet on the ground and slowly raise and lower the heels. If standing, perform as in heel raises but bend the knees.

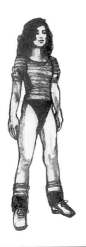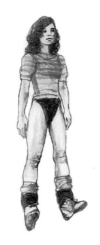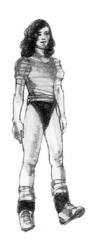

Foot lift

FOOT LIFT

major muscle used: **tibialis anterior (shin)**

Stand with your back against a wall, with your feet about 12 inches from the wall. Raise and lower your feet several times. You can raise your feet together and/or alternate them (21).

FOOT PRESS

major muscle used: **tibialis anterior**

Sit on the floor with your legs straight out in front of you. Have a partner sit in front of your legs and grasp both your feet; your toes should be pointed. Your partner applies downward pressure as you try to flex your ankle. Work through the full range of motion. Do not bend your knees. Repeat the exercise several times (21).

BODY TONING ROUTINES

Body toning and conditioning routines are made up of many of the exercises in this chapter combined with stretching exercises. Routines should involve all body parts, with smooth transitions from one exercise to the next. Two sample routines are described (p. 136). (Stretching exercises, which follow the body toning and conditioning phase, are described in Chapter 11.) You may vary your performance of the repetitions and counts of each exercise to fit your individual needs.

As the standing body toning routine becomes comfortable, you should repeat one and then two more sets of all the exercises as you simultaneously perform squats, lunges, or pliés so that you are working both the upper and lower body at the same time.

As these routines become easier, apply overload to add resistance and increase the difficulty by adding hand weights for the arms and ankle weights for the floor work. Place weights on the abdomen or chest to overload on the abdominal exercises. Use the step whenever possible to increase resistance and add variety to your workout.

FLOOR ROUTINE

Exercise	Repetitions	Counts
Curl-up	24	1 up, 1 down
Double curl	16	2 up, 2 down
Oblique curl	16 on each side	1 up, 1 down
Stretch arms and legs away from spine		32
Roll to stomach and with elbows on ground, arch up		32
Push-up	16, 2 down, 2 up	32
Chest stretch		32
Triceps stretch		32
Straight-leg lift	16 right, 16 left	1 up, 1 down
Bent-knee leg lift	16 right, 16 left	1 up, 1 down
Buttocks to heels stretch		32
Side thigh lift	16 right, 16 left	1 up, 1 down
Inner thigh lift	16 right, 16 left	1 up, 1 down
Pretzel stretch		32
Butterfly stretch		32

STANDING ROUTINE

Exercise	Repetitions	Counts
Lunges	8 right, 8 left	4 out, 4 in
Squats	8	4 down, 4 up
(Stay in squat position for the next exercises)		
Upright row	16	2 up, 2 down
Lateral arm raises	16	2 out, 2 in
Forward arm raises	16	2 up, 2 down
Upper back fly	16	2 out, 2 in
One-arm bent row	8 right, 8 left	2 out, 2 in
Triceps kickback	8 right, 8 left	2 out, 2 in
Biceps curl	16	2 up, 2 down

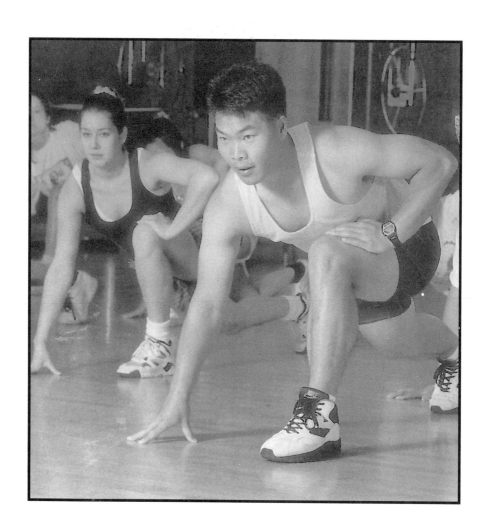

11

FLEXIBILITY AND STRETCHING

Stretching exercises are a part of the warm-up phase of the aerobic workout, as well as part of the final phase, the flexibility cool-down. Stretching during the warm-up

Increases the extensibility of the muscles

Reduces muscular resistance to rigorous physical exercise

Produces more efficient muscle contractions

Helps to reduce the chance of soreness or injury

Provides the psychological "readiness" to begin a workout program

Stretching in the warm-up may also include isolation exercises, which loosen and prepare isolated body parts for upcoming movement.

Stretching in the flexibility cool-down phase involves deep, static stretches, which minimize soreness but primarily serve to increase or maintain muscle and joint flexibility. Flexibility is a component of total fitness and is recommended as a conclusion to aerobic training by proponents of a well-rounded fitness philosophy.

Stretching exercises may be performed standing or lying. Generally, warm-up stretches are done standing and are integrated into the active warm-up. Standing stretches may also be performed at the conclusion of the aerobic cool-down. Floor stretches, however, are performed to emphasize increased range of motion. Floor stretches are of a longer duration and are the deep, static stretches used as the final phase of the aerobic workout.

It is important that flexibility exercises avoid awkward body positions and that the transitions between exercises be smooth. Careless stretching and improper technique can actually result in muscle tears and damage. Proper stretching technique is extremely important for the aerobic exercise.

PROPER STRETCHING TECHNIQUES

A long, sustained (static) stretch is best, rather than a bouncing (ballistic) stretch. Muscles have a stretch reflex; when you bounce, the reflex causes the muscles to react by tightening rather than by stretching.

When you are stretching, go to the point of mild tension. Relax in this position, and hold the stretch for 10 to 30 seconds. Release your position, and repeat the stretch. Before stretching a specific muscle, contract the opposing muscle. The reciprocal stretch exercise technique involves an isometric contraction of agonist muscles followed by a passive stretch of antagonist muscles of the same muscle group. For example, contract the quadriceps and then follow with a passive stretch of the hamstrings.

Always perform the exercises with proper body alignment. Two key areas of concern are the lower back and knees. Avoid holding your breath during any phase of an exercise; not breathing indicates a lack of relaxation. If your body vibrates or shakes during a stretch, ease up—you cannot relax if you are straining.

As you progress in the stretching exercises, keep in mind that flexibility is highly individual. Not all stretching exercises are appropriate for all people. Flexibility varies widely among people and also among the joints and muscles within each individual. Anatomical abnormalities or improperly performing an exercise can result in injury. If you perform an exercise correctly but experience abnormal pain, discontinue that particular exercise and seek professional advice regarding the problem.

The following section describes specific stretching exercises and their proper techniques.

STANDING STRETCHES

Neck

NECK ISOLATIONS

Drop your chin down. Tilt your head from side to side. Look to your right and left.

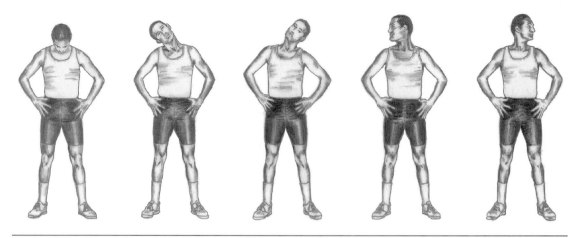

Neck isolations

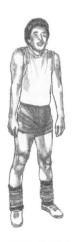
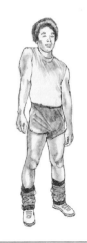

Shoulder shrugs

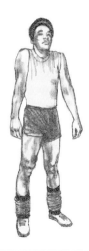

Shoulder circles

> ### ═ PRECAUTION ═
>
> *Head circles (not included in this text) have been identified as a contraindicated exercise; they can put undue stress on the cervical spine and should be avoided.*

Neck, Shoulders, Chest, and Arms

SHOULDER SHRUGS

Elevate your shoulders to your ears and then press your shoulders down. Lift both shoulders together and then one shoulder at a time.

SHOULDER CIRCLES

Because most people have a slight case of round shoulders due to desk work, housework, or other occupational situations, forward shoulder circles are not a necessary isolation exercise. Rather, to alleviate this problem, the isolation movement is performed in the backward direction. Be sure to go through the entire range of motion and use this exercise to relax the shoulder region.

CHEST STRETCH

muscles stretched: **pectoralis major
anterior deltoid**

Clasp your hands behind your back and stretch your chest muscles by pulling your shoulder blades together. You can also perform the chest stretch while bending forward at your waist and lifting your clasped hands away from your lower back, toward the ceiling.

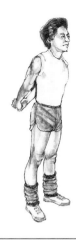

Chest stretch

SHOULDER AND RIB-CAGE PRESS

muscles stretched: **posterior deltoid
latissimus dorsi**

Stand in a straddle position, with your knees bent over your toes. Bend forward at

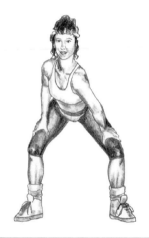

Shoulder and rib-cage press

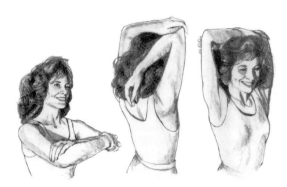

Elbow clasp over head

your hips and place your hands on your knees to support your upper body. Once you are in this position, slowly press one shoulder as far forward as possible. Hold the stretch, and then repeat it on the other side. This exercise not only stretches the shoulder girdle but also is beneficial in relieving compression in the lower back.

ELBOW CLASP OVER HEAD

muscle stretched: **triceps brachii**

Cross your arms in front of your body and hold your elbows with your hands. Raise your elbows overhead and pull back. For extra stretch, pull one elbow at a time. You can perform this exercise while standing, sitting, or kneeling.

BEHIND-THE-BACK TRICEPS STRETCH

muscle stretched: **triceps brachii**

This is another triceps stretch, performed behind the back, with your left arm over your head and your right arm gently stretching it by holding it at the upper arm or by the hand. Both versions of this stretch should be felt at the back of your arm and the upper parts of your shoulder and back. Repeat the stretch on your other side.

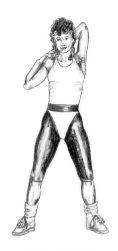

Behind-the-back triceps stretch

ACROSS-THE-BODY STRETCH

muscle stretched: **middle deltoid**

In a standing position with your feet shoulder width apart, or sitting cross-legged on the floor, keep your spine erect as you cross your right arm in front of your body and take hold of it with your left hand. Gently stretch your arm as close to your body as possible. Do not elevate your arm above your chest.

DELTOID ACROSS-CHEST OPPOSITION PULL

muscles stretched: **posterior deltoid**
                              latissimus dorsi

Start by standing in a straddle position, with your arms straight out in front of your chest, your left hand grasping your right wrist. Lunge onto your right leg, and pull your right arm across your chest to the left side of your body. Reverse the stretch to the opposite side. This is also an excellent stretch for the latissimus dorsi.

Torso

REACH STRETCH

muscles stretched: **latissimus dorsi**
                              external obliques

Reach up to the ceiling with one arm at a time. Fully stretch your side and rib cage. Do not hyperextend your rib cage or your lower back.

PRECAUTION

Because the aim of the reach stretch is to stretch the sides of the body, try not to elevate or tense the shoulders.

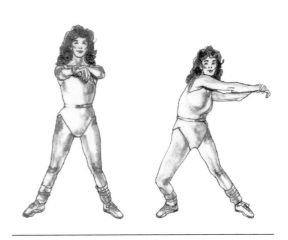

Deltoid across-chest opposition pull

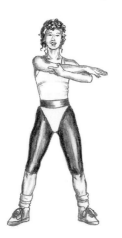

Across-the-body stretch

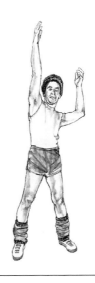

Reach stretch

HAND CLASP OVER HEAD

muscles stretched: **latissimus dorsi**
triceps brachii

Clasp your hands above your head and press your palms toward the ceiling, stretching your arms up and back. In this position, stretch to one side. Repeat the exercise to the other side. You can perform this exercise while standing, sitting, or kneeling. If standing, keep your knees relaxed.

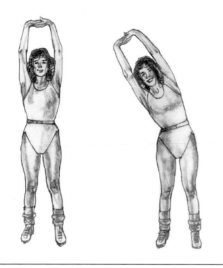

Hand clasp over head

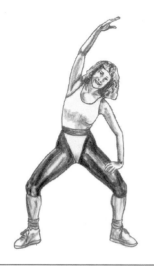

Lateral stretch

LATERAL STRETCH

muscles stretched: **latissimus dorsi**
triceps brachii

Stand with your feet shoulder width apart. Raise one arm over your head and bend *sideways* from your waist. Be sure you do not lean forward or backward; bend directly sideways. Do not move below your waist. To protect your lower back, support your trunk with your other hand on your thigh or your forearm on your thigh, keeping your knees slightly bent. You can perform this exercise with a variety of arm positions and from a sitting position.

PRECAUTIONS

- *Be sure to bend your knees slightly when performing this exercise.*
- *Contract your abdominals so that there is minimal stress on the lower back.*
- *Always support the stretch by placing one hand on your thigh.*

LUNGE WITH OVERHEAD OPPOSITION PULL

muscles stretched: **latissimus dorsi**
triceps brachii

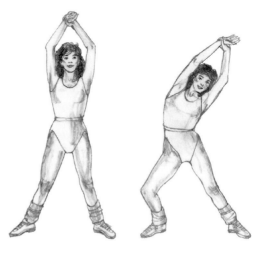

Lunge with overhead opposition pull

Start by standing in a straddle position, with your arms overhead, your left hand grasping your right wrist. Lunge onto your right leg, bending sideways at your waist to the left as your left arm pulls your right arm straight over your head. Reverse the stretch to the opposite side.

UPPER BACK STRETCH

muscles stretched: **rhomboids**
trapezius
erector spinae

In a standing position, with your feet shoulder width apart and your knees slightly bent, clasp your hands in front of your body and press your palms forward.

Another upper back stretch is to maintain the same standing position and wrap your arms around your body as if you were giving yourself a hug.

MOVEMENT TIPS

- *Keep the pelvis tucked under in this position so you can also feel the stretch at the lower back.*
- *Keep your abdominals tight while holding this stretch.*

Lower Body

KNEE-LIFT STRETCH

muscles stretched: **hamstrings**
gluteus maximus

Stand with your feet parallel and pull one knee to your chest, holding your leg underneath the thigh. You can also perform this stretch while lying on the floor with bent legs together. Pull one knee to your chest, holding your leg under the knee. This exercise stretches the hamstrings, gluteals, and lower back muscles.

PRECAUTIONS

- *In both positions, be sure to relax your supporting leg to alleviate any stress on the lower back.*
- *In both positions, attempt to maintain correct alignment.*

HAMSTRING STRETCH

muscles stretched: **hamstrings**
gastrocnemius
soleus

Stand with your feet shoulder width apart and extend one foot in front of the other in

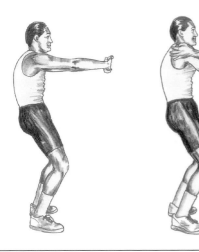

Upper back stretch

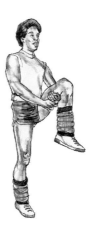

Knee-lift stretch

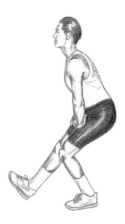

Hamstring stretch

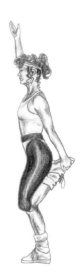

Standing quadriceps stretch

a parallel position. Bend your supporting leg and keep your front leg straight, with the foot flexed. Place both hands on your thighs for upper-body support.

PRECAUTIONS

- *Tighten your abdominals to relieve lower back strain.*
- *Do not hyperextend the straight leg.*
- *Keep your weight centered between your feet.*
- *Bend forward at the hip joint, keeping the spine neutral.*

MOVEMENT TIPS

- *Flex your foot as much as possible to achieve the maximum stretch.*
- *This stretch may also be performed on the step.*

STANDING QUADRICEPS STRETCH

muscles stretched: **quadriceps**
iliopsoas

You can perform this exercise in a variety of positions. The main idea is to bend your lower leg behind your body with the sole of your foot reaching toward the ceiling. Hold the lifted foot with your hand and stretch it toward your buttocks (refer to the *movement tips* following for additional positions).

MOVEMENT TIPS

- *You can do this exercise on the floor, lying either on your stomach with your leg pulled back or on your side with the top leg being stretched.*
- *For the less flexible individual, stand with your back to the wall. Place one foot against the wall, keeping your bent leg at a 90-degree angle.*
- *You can also perform this exercise with a partner, placing your free hand on the other person's shoulder for balance.*

PRECAUTIONS

- *If you feel pain in your bent knee, discontinue this exercise.*
- *Maintain proper alignment when performing this exercise.*

CALF STRETCH

muscles stretched: **gastrocnemius**
                                soleus
                                Achilles tendon

Stand with your feet together and parallel. Step with one foot forward so that your feet are approximately 1 to 2 feet apart. Lunge onto your front leg, being sure to keep your back leg straight and your back toes directed forward. Keep both heels on the floor. You can rest your hands on your front leg as an added weight to stretch your back leg.

PRECAUTIONS

- *The back heel must remain in contact with the floor in order to achieve the maximum stretch.*
- *Keep your bent knee in line with your ankle.*

MOVEMENT TIP

This stretch may also be performed using the step.

RUNNER LUNGE

muscles stretched: **iliopsoas**
                                gastrocnemius

From a deep lunge position, with your feet parallel, place your hands on the floor on either side of or on the inside of your forward, bent knee. In this position, the heel of your front foot must remain on the floor; your back leg should be straight with your foot fully flexed and your toes pressed against the floor.

PRECAUTIONS

Be sure your knee is directly over your ankle in this position. If your knee extends over or beyond your toes, there will be unnecessary stress on the knee ligament.

WIDE AND DEEP KNEE BEND

muscles stretched: **hip adductors**

Stand in a wide straddle position, with your legs turned out from your hip joints. Bend

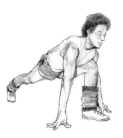

Runner lunge

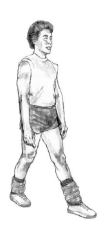 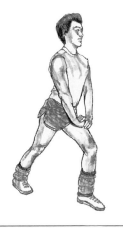

Calf stretch

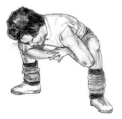

Wide and deep knee bend

deeply at your knees, keeping your heels flat on the ground. Press your thighs open with your elbows.

SIDE LUNGE

muscles stretched: **hip adductors**
gastrocnemius

Stand in a wide straddle position with your legs turned out from your hip joints and your hands on your thighs. Lunge by bending one knee and keeping your other leg straight. Make sure you do not compress your knee more than 90 degrees.

SOLEUS STRETCH

muscle stretched: **soleus**

Maintain the same standing position used for the calf stretch, but bend your back knee. Your back foot may be positioned closer to your front foot if necessary. Your back heel must remain on the ground. Your hands can be placed in any of the fundamental stretching positions.

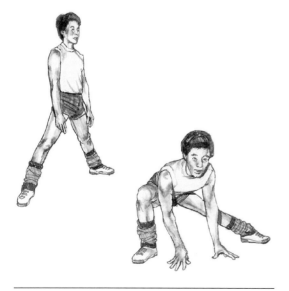

Side lunge

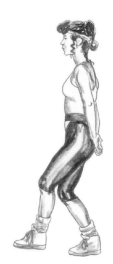

Soleus stretch

TOE TAP

muscle stretched: **tibialis anterior**

You can perform this exercise in many positions. In one common position, stand with your feet about 1 foot apart and your legs turned out from the hip joints. Tap your forward foot about 8 to 10 times and then repeat on the other side. You can also turn your foot out and in on alternating toe taps. This exercise warms up the shin muscle, tibialis anterior. The toe tap can also be performed in the runner lunge position as an added warm-up to the hip flexors.

Ankles

ANKLE FLEXION AND EXTENSION

muscles stretched: **tibialis anterior gastrocnemius**

Standing or sitting, flex (point your foot up) and then extend (point your foot down) your ankle slowly.

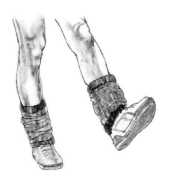

Ankle flexion

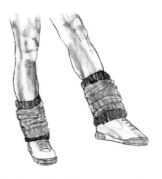

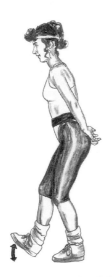

Toe tap

Ankle extension

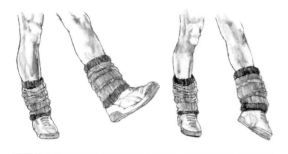

Ankle circle

ANKLE CIRCLES

Slowly circle your foot; be sure to circle in both directions. You can perform this exercise while standing or sitting.

FLOOR STRETCHES

Legs

FLOOR QUADRICEPS STRETCH

muscle stretched: **quadriceps**

In a side-lying or front-lying position, bend the leg and grasp the ankle. Pull the heel of the foot toward the buttocks. Turn to the other side and repeat with the other leg.

> **PRECAUTION**
>
> *If you feel pain in the bent knee, discontinue this exercise.*

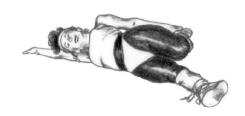

Floor quadriceps stretch

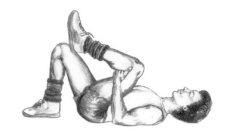

Knee to chest

KNEE TO CHEST

muscles stretched: **hamstrings**
                    gluteus maximus

Lying on your back, pull one knee to your chest, holding your thigh under the knee. Pull the thigh to your chest.

> **PRECAUTIONS**
>
> • *The nonstretching leg should be bent, foot firmly placed on floor to help secure correct hip placement.*
> • *Contract the abdominals, pressing the lumbar spine against the floor, to reduce risk of lower back strain.*
> • *Do not grasp the leg over the knee; this may cause undue stress on the knee joint.*

GLUTEAL STRETCH

muscles stretched: **gluteus maximus**
                   hip adductors
                   gluteus medius
                   gluteus minimus

Lying on your back, start with your knees bent and the soles of your feet on the ground. Cross your right ankle onto your left thigh. Pull your knees to your chest by grasping your left thigh. Repeat this stretch on your left leg.

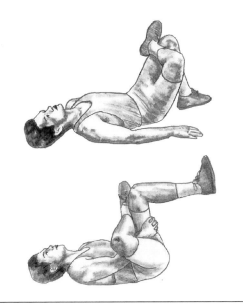

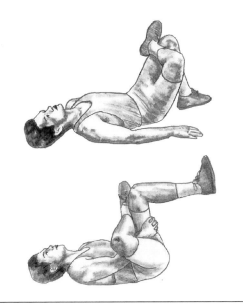

Gluteal stretch

PELVIC TILT

muscles stretched: **rectus abdominus
iliopsoas**

Lie on your back, with your knees bent, the soles of your feet on the floor, and your hands at your sides. Tightening your buttocks, lift your hips toward the ceiling, approximately 2 inches off the floor. Release

the stretch, lowering your back and hips to the floor one vertebra at a time. The pelvic tilt also stretches the thigh and abdominal muscles. *Note:* The pelvic tilt may be done as a body toning exercise by advanced students who understand the body concept of tightening the gluteus and abdominal muscles to support the lower back. As a body toning and conditioning exercise, the pelvic tilt is done repeatedly in more rapid succession and works to tone and condition the gluteus muscle.

INDIAN SIT GLUTEAL STRETCH

muscles stretched: **hip adductors**

Sitting with your back straight, cross your legs Indian style. Keep both your hips in contact with the floor. Reverse the cross of your legs to stretch both hips equally. Isolations, rib cage and torso exercises, and arm movements may be performed in this position.

BUTTERFLY STRETCH

muscles stretched: **gluteus maximus
hip adductors**

Sitting with your back straight, bring the soles of your feet together, with your knees bent. Hold your ankles, and press your pelvic girdle forward, keeping your back straight. Gently press your knees toward the floor to increase the flexibility of your hip joints.

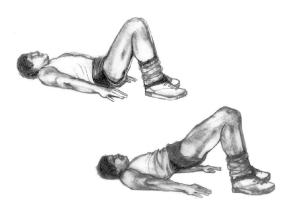

Pelvic tilt

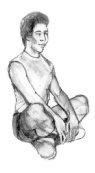

Indian sit gluteal stretch

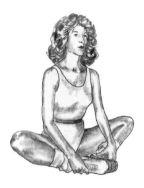

Butterfly stretch

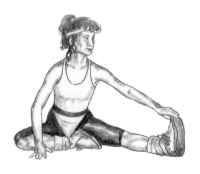

Foot-to-groin straddle stretch

MODIFIED PRETZEL

muscles stretched: **hip abductors**
gluteus maximus
gluteus medius

Sitting with your back straight, cross your legs Indian style. Straighten your left leg and place your right foot on the outside of your left thigh. Keep your back straight, and pull your right knee toward your chest with your left arm while pressing your hip toward the floor. Reverse the stretch to your left leg.

FOOT-TO-GROIN STRADDLE STRETCH

muscles stretched: **hamstring**
gastrocnemius
hip adductors
hip abductors

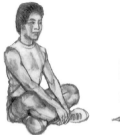
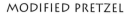

Modified pretzel

Bend your right leg so that your right foot touches your groin. Relax the trunk of your body over your left leg. Repeat the stretch on your right leg.

> ### PRECAUTION
>
> *A groin stretch, commonly called the* hurdler's stretch *(one leg is bent so that the foot touches the buttocks while the trunk of the body stretches forward over an extended leg), can gradually stretch the ligaments on the inside of the knee (medial collateral ligament) and the tissue of the groin, causing painful fascial groin pulls.*

STARTING POSITION FOR STRADDLE STRETCH

muscles stretched: **hip adductors**
hip abductors

Sitting with your back straight, open your legs as wide as possible to a straddle position. Your hips will remain on the floor, and your knees will face the ceiling on the straddle side stretch.

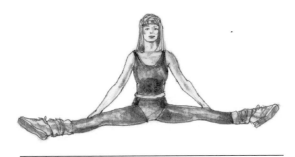

Starting position for straddle stretch

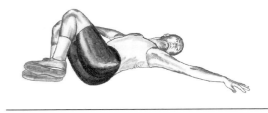

Spinal rotation

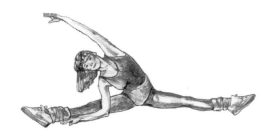

Straddle side stretch

PRECAUTIONS

- *Do not let your legs roll forward. Keep your knees rotated toward the ceiling.*
- *Keep your knees relaxed.*
- *Do not allow either buttock to lift from the floor.*

Back

SPINAL ROTATION

muscles stretched: **obliques**
erector spinae

Lie on your back, with your knees bent to your chest and your arms extended out to the sides at shoulder height. Drop your knees to the right, and look at your left hand. Keep both shoulders on the floor, and relax in this position. Repeat on the other side. For individuals with back problems, keep your feet on the floor while lowering your knees to the side.

PRECAUTIONS

- *Do not arch your back.*
- *Do not hold your breath.*

STRADDLE SIDE STRETCH

muscles stretched: **hip adductors**
latissimus dorsi

Place your right arm from your elbow to your palm on the floor, either inside or outside your right leg. Your left arm reaches overhead while you are stretching your right leg. Reverse the stretch toward your left leg.

CAT STRETCH

muscle stretched: **erector spinae**

Begin on your hands and knees. Contract your rib cage and stomach; keep your head down. Curve your spine and hold this position for 10 seconds. Return your chest and back to a neutral position before repeating the exercise. To achieve maximum results, it is important to contract your abdominal muscles.

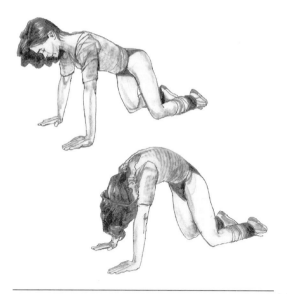

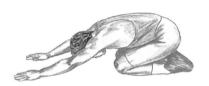

Cat stretch

Buttocks-to-heels reach stretch

PRECAUTION

- *Do not arch your lower back or sag in your abdominal region in the starting position.*
- *Do not lock your elbows.*

BUTTOCKS-TO-HEELS REACH STRETCH

muscles stretched: **gluteus maximus**
trapezius
latissimus dorsi

Kneeling on the floor, keep your buttocks as close to your heels as possible. Relax your upper body over your thighs, and reach your arms forward along the floor.

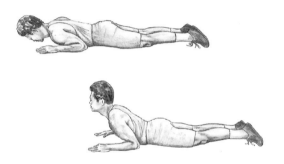

Low cobra

This exercise is excellent for relieving stress in the lower back as well as stretching the chest, shoulder, and triceps muscles.

Abdominals

ABDOMINAL STRETCH

muscle stretched: **rectus abdominus**

Lying on your back, stretch your arms overhead while stretching your legs and flexing your feet. This stretch is effective immediately after abdominal strengthening and endurance exercises.

LOW COBRA

muscles stretched: **rectus abdominus**
pectoralis major

Lying prone on the floor, place your hands on the floor near your shoulders. Keeping your elbows on the floor, lift your chest off the floor and arch your upper back. Keep your hips down and lower back relaxed. Slowly bend your arms to lower your chest to the starting position. Do several rhythmic repetitions.

PRECAUTION

For the low cobra avoid the "swan" version (overarched lower back position) of this exercise, which places excessive hypertension in the lumbar area.

STRETCH ROUTINES

FLOOR STRETCH ROUTINE

Steps

1. Begin lying on the back*
2. Knee to chest stretch right
3. Gluteal stretch (cross right leg on top)
4. Knee to chest stretch left
5. Gluteal stretch (cross left leg on top)
6. Pelvic tilt
7. Floor quadriceps stretch right leg, left leg
8. Low cobra
9. Buttocks-to-heel reach stretch
10. Cat stretch
11. Sit: butterfly stretch
12. Foot-to-groin straddle stretch right
13. Foot-to-groin straddle stretch left
14. Modified pretzel, right and left

Note: The counts to music are not as important as the time length of each stretch. Warm-up stretches should be approximately 10 seconds each. Deep flexibility stretches featured in this routine, which is designed for the end of class, can be as long as 30 seconds for each stretch.

STANDING STRETCH ROUTINE

Steps	*Counts*
Begin with feet shoulder width apart	
1. Neck isolation (look right and left)	8
2. Shoulder and rib-cage press (2 counts each: right, left, right, left)	8
3. Deltoid across-chest (4 counts right arm, 4 counts left arm)	8
4. Reach stretch (1 count each reach, alternating arms)	8
5. Lateral stretch (4 counts right arm, 4 counts left arm)	8
6 Upper back stretch	8
7. Knee lift stretch right	8
8. Knee lift stretch left	8
9. Standing quadriceps stretch right	8
10. Standing quadriceps stretch left	
11. Calf stretch right	8
12. Calf stretch left	8
13. Soleus stretch right	8
14. Soleus stretch left	8

RELAXATION

Relaxation exercises are a good follow-up to flexibility floor exercises. The relaxation phase of a workout is not always included in the aerobics class. However, relaxation is often a welcome conclusion to the workout. The relaxation phase can be a possible tool for managing stress.

Symptoms of abnormal states of stress include restlessness, lack of concentration, tension, anxiety, unreasonable irritability and depression, headaches, insomnia, nightmares, depressed appetite, or increased smoking (7). Everyone occasionally experiences one or more of these states, but it is not normal to be continually beset with them. There are many passive and active techniques to help individuals manage stress. For some of us, relaxation is a skill we must acquire. In our complex world, a life totally devoid of stress is nearly impossible, but by taking the time and making a conscious effort, we can achieve the ability to relax. To quote the poet Ovid: "What is without periods of rest will not endure."

Passive Relaxation Techniques

Passive relaxation techniques include total relaxation, meditation, and visual imagery. A quiet room with minimal distractions is necessary for following through with these mental relaxation techniques.

Total Relaxation Lie on your back in a comfortable position. Take a deep breath, counting to 5 when you inhale; count to 10 when you exhale. Focus your concentration on this breathing pattern, mentally dismissing all outside distractions. As you continue, begin to form a mental image of how you look when you are relaxed: Your jaw has dropped; your neck is loose; your eyes are drowsy; your legs, hips, and back are heavy. Your breathing is light and easy. Continue this exercise for at least 5 to 10 minutes to experience a state of total relaxation.

Meditation Sit in a cross-legged position, resting your hands in your lap or on your knees. Close your eyes and totally relax all your muscles. Concentrate on a simple, single word or sound while breathing slowly and rhythmically. If your mind drifts, refocus your thoughts back to the word or sound. Continue thinking of that one word or sound for about 20 minutes. When you finish, sit quietly for several minutes with your eyes open. Then stand up slowly.

Visual Imagery Lie on your back and get as comfortable as possible. Close your eyes and begin to build a serene world in your mind, such as a mountain lake with the sun shining and a warm breeze blowing. Visualize every detail of the scene, and place yourself in this environment. Continue this visualization for at least 10 minutes. Open your eyes and sit quietly for several minutes. Then stand up slowly.

Active Relaxation Techniques

Find a warm, quiet space with as few distractions as possible. Your body must be in a relaxed position. For the sitting position, rest your hands on your thighs, with your fingers spread, head hung gently forward, and all your muscles

relaxed. For the lying position, lie on a bed or the floor. Spread your legs, let your feet point away from your body, place your arms away from the sides of your body with your palms down and fingers spread. For added support, you can place a pillow or rolled towel under your neck, at the curve in your lower back, and under your knees and elbows (35). Give yourself at least 10 minutes to complete the following exercises in a relaxed manner.

Progressive Relaxation The goal of this technique is to achieve the sensation of complete muscular relaxation after experiencing complete muscular tension.

First lie on your back with your legs straight and your hands at the sides of your body. Relax as best you can.

Next, contract your facial muscles by tightly closing your eyes and clenching your teeth, keeping your mouth tightly closed. Release the tension slowly to the count of 10.

Clench your fist as hard as you can and hold the position for 5 seconds and feel the tension. Feel the tension in your arm? Release the tension very slowly to the count of 10. Repeat this exercise with your other arm.

Flex your feet and tighten the quadriceps muscles in each leg. Hold the tension for 5 seconds and feel the tension. Release slowly to the count of 10. Repeat this tension and relaxation process by tightening and releasing your buttock and stomach muscles.

Slow, Controlled Movements for Your Head and Torso Slow, controlled movements or large, rhythmical, free-flowing movements also help promote relaxation. Sit on the floor or in a chair in a comfortable position so that you feel no undue muscular tension. Breathe slowly and rhythmically when performing the following movements.

Perform slow, easy neck swings; do not swing your head to the back. Now perform slow, easy shoulder circles. Next, perform slow, easy side bends with your spine, keeping your arms relaxed at your sides. Relax your spine forward and breathe easily.

Exercise can also be a tool for releasing daily tension and increasing your ability to understand stressful conditions. Although experts cannot agree about exactly how exercise works this way, various theories suggest that exercise may simply be a diversion, freeing the mind from stresses that contribute to anxiety (1); that a feeling of accomplishment (of a physical goal) is a factor (2); and that exercise reduces muscular tension, thus inducing a state of muscular relaxation (3). If you exercise to help reduce stress, you must not overexercise, which will recreate a state of stress.

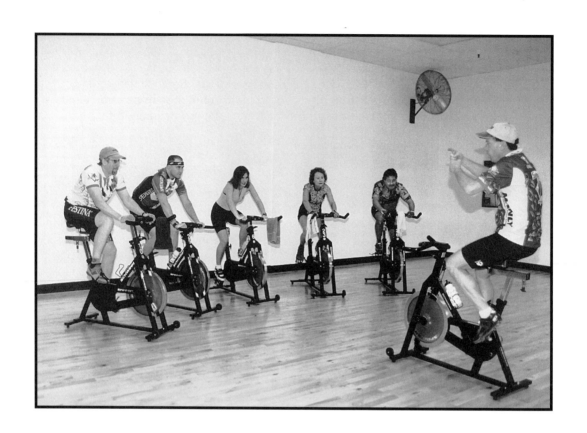

12

ADDING VARIETY TO YOUR AEROBIC WORKOUT

As you become regularly involved in an aerobics program, you may want to explore the variety of alternative aerobics programs available. By adding variety to your aerobic conditioning program, you will add interest to your training regime, keeping yourself enthusiastic and motivated. Although each program has virtually the same aerobic training foundation, each activity emphasizes a slightly different set of muscles used or may vary in building the areas of strength, flexibility, or endurance. More and more fitness educators and trainers believe that *cross-training*, or diversity in a training program, increases total fitness, reduces overuse injuries, and is an antidote to exercise burnout.

Included in this chapter are descriptions of some of the programs you may wish to explore to add variety to your workout routine.

FUNK AEROBICS/ CARDIOFUNK

When your regular aerobics class seems to be too familiar, too straight up, too stiff—why not give a little soulful oomph a try? In funk aerobics, many of the common aerobics steps are the same, only done with what funk aerobicizers call "attitude." For instance, the grapevine, so common a step in aerobics classes, can be changed to a funky alternative. Funk it up with a shoulder isolation, add a little nod of the head forward and back in time with the music, and finish the step with a quick knee lift and twist. And don't forget to loosen up those hips! Remember part of funk is attitude and understated cool.

CardioFunk also combines flashy MTV-type dance movements with the usual aerobics movements. A variety of street-style jazz moves are included, as opposed to the more athletic movements used in regular aerobic workouts. Funk aerobics includes a combination of dance steps: jazz steps and movements, funk, hip-hop, and rap. Funk aerobics uses club music, pop, funk, rap, and soul to make funk more hip-hopping, bebopping, and dance oriented.

Hand movements and facial expression convey a sense of personal freedom and creativity. In funk, students are encouraged to move in a way that is comfortable for them, concentrating on the music and letting their bodies move to the beat.

YOGAEROBICS

Yogaerobics combines aerobics with the techniques of yoga and the movement of tai chi. The aerobics portion of the class is the driving energy force of the class while the yoga instruction helps to soothe and balance mind and body. Classes begin with the stillness of meditation and yoga stretches, progressing through lyrical movements, as well as the circular movements of tai chi. Continual movement throughout each phase of the workout helps to increase cardiorespiratory endurance.

The music used in the class is not the typical pop music common to the aerobics industry. Much of the music is Eastern-influenced sounds, tinkling and swirling sounds that move the body continuously and fluidly. Percussion instruments can also lead the class, the music of a tribal beat prompting movements for high-intensity endurance. The final phase of the class is the return to the original stillness of yoga. Yogaerobics students feel that this type of aerobic exercise is the true blending of body, mind, and spirit. After completing a Yogaerobics class, participants feel not only vitalized and full of energy but also mentally balanced and centered.

BOXING-BASED AEROBIC PROGRAMS

A new trend in aerobic training is boxing workouts with names like Boxercise, Boxerobics, Cardio Knockout, and other hard-hitting pseudonyms. The boxing workout is an intense cardiorespiratory training program with upperbody strengthening and conditioning. It is the convergence of a number of fitness disciplines—primarily boxing, aerobics, and circuit training. Boxing provides the background for the workout and aims at all-over physical conditioning.

The boxing workout normally lasts an hour and is led by a specialist instructor using professional boxing equipment. As in all aerobic-type classes, the session begins with the warm-up. The boxing warm-up uses gentle aerobic and anaerobic exercise with calisthenic exercises. Following the warm-up is the boxing workout, which includes strength training, rope jumping, shadow boxing, and punching a bag or focus mitt. The workout includes several circuits, each consisting of a number of *rounds*. The time and intensity of the round depend on the participant's skill and fitness levels. A round begins with low-impact exercise lasting 10 to 30 seconds, advances to mid-impact exercise lasting 30 to 60 seconds, and ends with high-impact activity lasting 1 to 2 minutes. Also included in the rounds are shadow-boxing drills, bag drills, and one-on-one training, that is, working with a partner (involving no contact with the opponent other than a trainer's focus mitt).

The boxing workout ends with a cool-down and stretch. The cool-down includes additional exercises for strength and toning. Extra time is allowed for the stretching portion of the class. The stretch-out emphasizes exercises for muscle suppleness and is targeted for performance improvement and injury prevention.

Participants in boxing-based aerobic programs feel the benefits of this training workout are varied. Workout benefits include improvement in cardiovascular fitness as well as muscular strength and tone. Many students cite a reduction in stress as well as greater confidence. Women, in particular, appreciate the benefits of a training program that not only emphasizes all the aspects of fitness training but also makes them feel less like a potential victim. Participants feel more fit, safer, and in greater control of their own well-being.

MARTIAL–ARTS–BASED AEROBIC PROGRAMS

Students not ready to commit to a regimented martial arts training program can find a popular alternative in aerobic martial arts classes. These classes go by many names: cardio-karate, karatics, kempocise, Tae-Bo, TKO Aerobics, and many more, although they are generally referred to as aerobic kickboxing. Students in aerobic kickboxing classes have a different agenda and goals than regular martial arts students; kickboxing students want to gain cardio-fitness benefits and feel good about their bodies rather than attain belt levels associated with the martial arts. Yet many benefits of martial arts training, such as self-defense techniques and discipline, naturally develop as kickboxing students progress in their training.

As in other aerobics classes, the kickboxing class is set to music. The warm-up includes jogging, jumping jacks, calisthenics, and sometimes jumping rope, to warm the body and elevate the heart rate. Toward the end of the warm-up, students do power stretching and may do special yoga stretches, depending on which martial art the program is based on. Punches and kicks warm up arms and legs for the next part of the workout, which involves basic self-defense techniques.

Punching techniques such as cross punches, upper cuts, and hook punches are all done with the legs bent and stances low. Basic punches are followed by jabs, and combinations of jabs and punches. Students continue with punching techniques while beginning to move and travel. Students begin to jump, first jumping without switching legs, then jumping while switching forward and back legs. All the time, students are punching with each movement.

Kicking exercise may begin easily, using knee lifts as a way to warm up the hip joint and its surrounding muscles. Simple kicks, such as the front kick, the side kick, and the roundhouse kick, begin the series of kicking drills. More intensive kicking techniques include jump kicking from a squatting position, or machine-gun kicks, which are jumping roundhouse or side kicks that continue without stopping.

Other training drills included in the workout may be speed bag drills, done both with and without the bag. These drills develop better speed, upper-body muscle tone, and hand-eye coordination. Aerobic kickboxers also shadow box to lively music using special patterns such as standing straight, then stepping forward to execute a kick, and then delivering a series of punching techniques.

Throughout the kickboxing workout, instructors teach proper punching, kicking, and self-defense techniques as well as the purpose of each technique. Correct form in executing movements is essential for avoiding potential injury.

The intensive kickboxing workout returns to a moderate pace with a cool-down using hanging or free-standing bags, or focus pads. Cool-down exercises may include 10 minutes of apparatus training involving skill combinations of kicking and punching actions. During the apparatus part of the workout, students wear boxing gloves. Also included in the cool-down are body toning exercises. Sit-ups, push-ups, and leg exercises are all part of the toning phase. Deep stretching ends the workout session with an emphasis on flexibility, an integral part of any martial arts program.

There is no question that aerobic kickboxing is a great way to improve cardiovascular and muscular fitness. Classes are designed to develop all parts of the body equally. And the workout burns anywhere from 400 to 800 calories per hour! As well as improved fitness, students develop basic self-defense techniques and a knowledge that they can defend themselves. All in all, students gain both physically and mentally.

Instructors agree that, no matter what name it goes by, there is an overwhelming amount of enthusiasm for the aerobic kickboxing workout.

JUMP ROPE

The simple childhood activity of skipping rope has made its way into the aerobics world. Several commercial videos can help a student learn the proper way to jump rope, beginning with simple drills to help timing and coordination of jumping and skipping in time with the rope motion. These drills help synchronize upper- and lower-body timing before going into a workout of rope jumping. Good form is essential to minimize possible injury to the ankles, knees, and lower back. Common mistakes are jumping stiff-legged or kicking up the heels.

Jump ropes are often used in classes that are geared to athletic training. Some popular new names for these classes are "boot camp" or "fit camp." These athletic training classes use such common jump-rope exercises as jumping in place, which requires the student to rebound quickly between jumps. Another common jump-rope exercise is standing jumps; large single jumps with full recovery between jumps. Both of these jumping techniques can also be performed as hops. Multiple jumps and hops are combinations of jumping in place and standing jumps. Other jumping exercises include box jumps and bounding jumps. Box-jumping drills incorporate jumping both forward and backward and side to side. Bounding-jump exercises exaggerate the normal running stride as a way to improve both stride length and quickness.

Jump ropes are used not only to improve athletic skills that involve jumping but also as a way to increase aerobic and anaerobic endurance. Jumping at a steady pace burns about the same number of calories as running but has less impact because, when jumping properly, the feet barely lift off the ground. For cardiorespiratory endurance, 10 minutes of jumping is claimed to be as effective as 10 minutes of running.

SLIDE AEROBICS

Slide aerobics is a type of conditioning program in which a slide board is used to perform the aerobic movements and exercises. Slide aerobics, or the slide, looks like skating in place, as the exerciser glides side to side on a slide board, which is a stationary piece of slick material. Nylon booties are fitted over a pair of athletic shoes (aerobics shoes, cross-trainers, or court shoes provide good lateral support). Students keep their hands in front of the body for balance as the body leans slightly forward.

The slide board is known in the exercise science industry as a lateral movement trainer. The lateral trainer was first used in rehabilitation for torn anterior cruciate ligaments of the knee. However, the popularity of the slide has exploded because of its effective training of the cardiorespiratory system with the advantage of nonimpact exercise. The push-off phase requires the use of major large muscle groups: the whole hip extensor group of the gluteus muscles and the knee extensor group of the quadriceps, as well as the gastrocnemius and soleus. The lateral motion of the slide involves the hip adductors and hip abductors. To overcome the inertia of the sliding phase, the hamstrings are in a contraction throughout the slide. Finally to maintain the forward bent position and to maintain balance, the postural muscles, mainly the back extensors and the abdominals, are used.

The aerobic benefits of the slide are many. However, success in using the slide depends largely on the instruction of the class leader. The surface of the slide board is slick and caution should be used. The power needed for the push-off will take several repetitions to learn. Once mastered, the slide is an inexpensive, portable, and fun way to obtain a demanding aerobic workout.

GROUP INDOOR CYCLE

Group indoor cycling programs combine a foundation of basic cycling movements with heart rate training, breathing awareness, and motivational coaching techniques led by a certified instructor. Indoor cycling programs have been developed by a variety of aerobic certification groups such as Body Bike, Cycle Reebok, Keiser Power Pacer, and Johnny G Spinning.

Indoor cycling programs utilize a stationary bike designed to simulate a real outdoor bicycling experience. Bikes have racing handlebars; pedals with clips or cages; a seat that can be adjusted up and down, forward and backward; a resistance knob that can be used to adjust the resistance of the flywheel; and a water-bottle cage. Both men and women participate in the program; its appeal crosses both genders because it emulates a bike ride. When weather or time does not permit a long bike ride, participants can take a cycling class and ride through imaginary terrain in less than an hour, and they can get aerobic training benefits similar to those of an outdoor ride. During the cycling workout the instructor talks the class through the imaginary ride, coaching each participant with visualization and motivational techniques to help achieve the workout goals. A variety of background music helps set the pace of the ride and also helps to inspire participants.

Appropriate attire helps make the class more enjoyable. Bicycle shorts have an antibacterial moisture-wicking pad, which also helps alleviate the discomfort of the bicycle seat. Bicycle shirts also help to wick perspiration, although a T-shirt could be worn. Heart rate monitors are also encouraged, because exercise heart rate is used to measure workout intensity.

There are different heart rate training zones depending upon the class format. The lower heart rate training zones promote active recovery and fat burning. The middle heart rate zones are for increasing endurance and aerobic capacity. The higher heart rate zones increase the rider's ability to raise his/her anaerobic threshold. The highest heart rate zones are reserved for maximum efforts like sprinting. When choosing the level of intensity for your workout, it is important to be aware of the class format. Group indoor cycling class formats may have a variety of names, but basically programs include classes for endurance workouts, strength workouts, all-terrain workouts, and recovery workouts.

Endurance workouts are at a heart rate training range of 65 to 75 percent of the maximum. An endurance workout promotes the most consistent usage of energy. The emphasis is on finding the optimum cycling pace that can be maintained for an extended period of time. The cycling must be strenuous enough to raise the heart rate into the target zone between 65 to 75 percent. The goal of the endurance workout is to increase aerobic capacity and resist fatigue. Increased aerobic capacity translates into longer durations than an individual is able to maintain at a pace that is in the 65 to 75 percent target training zone.

Strength workouts are at a heart rate training range of 75 to 85 percent. The strength workout is performed at a slow, steady pace with a high level of resistance. Most strength training in cycling is done in the hills and requires specific leg muscular power as well as aerobic endurance. To simulate the feeling of "climbing a hill," resistance on the wheel of the bike is increased gradually and constantly. Pacing on the hill climb is important, and participants must constantly monitor their heart rate to keep within 75 to 85 percent of the maximum. The goal of this ride simulation is to keep "climbing up the hill" for the length of the workout. Recovery from this workout is critical.

The *all-terrain* workout covers the entire aerobic training zone from 65 to 90 percent and also includes anaerobic work up to 92 percent. An all-terrain workout utilizes a variety of cycling skills. The ride simulates cycling on the flats, hills, acceleration drills (sprinting), jumps, and recovery pace riding. Riders train at each intensity level, and the sprint workout is used to train riders anaerobically. Heart rate monitoring is essential as the instructor leads the class through the variety of cycling training drills. Riders must monitor the heart rate to be at the proper intensity level and training zone depending on the phase of the workout and cycling skill being utilized.

The *recovery* workout is in the heart rate training range of 50 to 65 percent of the maximum. Passive recovery is taking a day off. Active recovery is a light workout that has been found to actually help the body's recovery process. The recovery workout helps to rejuvenate the body, and the ride focuses on balance, breathing, and centering the psyche. Visualization includes energy accumulation in the body. The workout should be kept at a light resistance level on the wheel, and it is important to stay within 50 to 65 percent of the heart rate training zone.

Indoor cycling is simple, fun, and easy to learn. It is a low-impact sport, so it does not impose great stress on the body and its joints. Regardless of age, size, or fitness level, anyone can do it!

WATER FITNESS CLASSES

Water fitness, or aqua aerobics, is not simply a land aerobics class set in the pool. However, its format is very similar to other aerobics classes. The warm-up for this class begins either on deck or in the pool. The class builds to a full aerobic workout, eases into an aerobic cool-down and muscle toning session, and finally finishes with a flexibility stretching session. The workout is set to motivating music, is in a cool environment, and has little to no impact stress.

The unique properties of water affect exercise intensity and influence movements, because the water supplies a natural resistance. The water's resistance challenges the body's ability to overcome inertia, and any movement changes will increase intensity. Starting and stopping a movement (walking forward to in-place marching) require more energy than continuing a movement (walking forward only). Changing movement direction (jog forward, then jog backward) requires more energy than continuing a movement direction. By using the water effectively in the manner described here, participants can increase exercise intensity and elevate heart rates.

Monitoring exercise intensity using the target heart rate may be influenced by factors inherent to the aquatic medium. Because the body cools four times faster in water than on land, it may be easier for the body to get rid of excess heat. The result of this effect is a lower exercising heart rate. The Cooper Institute suggests deducting 17 beats per minute from target heart rates when exercising in the water. Take this variable into account when calculating the target heart rate for aqua aerobics. Although heart rates in water fitness classes tend to be lower than in land classes, th. metabolic and cardiovascular benefits are comparable.

Balanced muscles workouts can be easily achieved in the aqua aerobics class, because water resistance is experienced through the entire range of motion of any part of the body being used. For example, water impedes movement during the biceps curl equally as much as it impedes movement during arm extensions or the triceps press. Because both agonist and antagonist muscle groups are continually working against resistance, muscle strength and endurance are balanced in their development throughout the full aquatic workout.

Pool attire for the aqua aerobics class may seem obvious, but there are a few tips to consider. If you chill easily, wear tights or a leotard in the pool. Specialty snorkeling or scuba "skins" are the same as a lycra unitard and can also alleviate chill. Aqua shoes can help prevent foot abrasions caused by pushing off the pool bottom, provide cushioning for the balls of the feet, and supply traction for the pool bottom and deck.

Some aqua classes may use equipment such as balls, webbed gloves, and plastic or foam hand weights. Such apparatus are typically used during the body toning phase of the class. For deep-water work, there are flotation belts, jogging vests, kick boards, and other devices to provide buoyancy and support for your body. The tether, another training tool, provides resistance for sports-specific training.

As aqua aerobics has grown in popularity, it has branched out to include a variety of workout formats. Some classes resemble aerobic dance exercise, some use weighted step boxes for aqua step aerobics, some include strictly deep-water running exercises, and some use circuit- and interval-type training principles. Anyone of any age and fitness level can do aqua aerobics. It can also be easily modified for people of varying fitness levels to participate in the same class. Aqua aerobics—take the plunge!

TRAINING PROGRAMS

All of the alternative aerobic workouts just described can be altered and combined in training programs such as interval training, circuit training, and cross-training. These methods of conditioning have been used to train athletes for many years. Recently, these methods have been implemented in aerobics classes as an alternative to the standard class format.

Interval Training

Interval training is a series of high-intensity exercises alternated with periods of light- or mild-intensity exercise. Because the intensity of training is not continuous, the workload and the demand on the cardiorespiratory system can be overloaded (90 to 100 percent capacity). By altering the intensity of the training and by al-

lowing the body a small phase of recovery during the training, the body is able to adjust to the more intense workload.

The important terms that define an interval training program are listed below:

> *Work interval*—this is the high-intensity workload portion of the workout. The body works at the high end of its target heart range. It should last no more than 90 seconds.

> *Rest interval*—this segment follows the work interval. During this phase, the body works at the lowest end of its target heart range. The rest interval usually lasts twice as long as the work interval.

An interval training workout involves a period of high-intensity exercises interspersed with rest intervals. The work interval consists of grouped exercises (*sets*), a number of exercises per set (*repetitions*), and resting time between repetitions, or as we have defined it, the rest interval.

So how can interval training be used for the aerobic workout? After the warm-up, begin with the rest interval, a pre-aerobic phase using mild exercise to progressively increase the heart rate. Or begin with the work interval, as an aerobic phase. In either situation, the work interval should use high-intensity movements such as hops, jumps, and leaps, allowing the heart rate to achieve 90 to 100 percent of its maximum. The work interval should be followed by a rest interval using movements such as walking, marching, light jogging, or other low-impact or nonimpact aerobic movements. The length and time of the work and rest intervals can vary depending upon the ability of the participants. But in order to improve the aerobic energy system, a minimum ratio of 1:2 time length for the work/rest intervals is necessary. Gradually decrease the rest interval to a ratio of 1:1, and then further to $1:\frac{1}{2}$ to continue to improve cardiorespiratory endurance.

Interval training is not appropriate for the beginner. It is best suited to the aerobic student who needs to increase the intensity of his or her current workout or who wants variety in his or her present exercise regime.

Circuit Training

Circuit training is not new. However, aerobic circuit training has now become a widely popular class format for aerobics enthusiasts. **Circuit training** consists of a number of "stations," where a specific exercise or routine is performed in a given period of time. Once the exercise is completed, the participant moves quickly to the next station, also performed in a specific time frame. Once all the stations have been completed, the circuit is finished. Aerobic circuit training combines aerobic exercise (to build cardiorespiratory endurance) with weight-training exercises (to develop muscular strength and endurance). By alternating aerobic and weight-training exercise stations, this combined workout can provide maximum benefits.

It is important that the sequencing of exercises in a circuit be arranged so that no two consecutive stations work the same muscle group. By placing aerobic stations between the stations, you develop your cardiovascular endurance as well as muscular endurance. However, to maintain the elevated heart rate achieved at the aerobic stations, you must move quickly from one station to the next. It is also important that strength-training exercises be performed at an "aerobic" pace, using light weights and quick repetitions. The emphasis on weight-training work is to develop muscular endurance rather than power or strength.

The format for an aerobic circuit training session is based on timed intervals at each station, which will be determined by your instructor. Each station usually takes 45 to 75 seconds. You attempt to do as many repetitions as you can within that time slot. After completing that station, you go to the next one directly, or when the instructor calls "change."

Another method for integrating an aerobic circuit program into an aerobics class is to perform 10 minutes of aerobics with the group and then complete a muscular strength or muscular endurance circuit for 10 minutes. Repeat this sequence for the length of the class. In both methods, be sure to warm up and cool down!

One of the many advantages of aerobic circuit training is the versatility of the program. Students may work with a class, individually, or in a buddy system—with another classmate or the instructor. Workout programs can be tailored to meet individual goals by making different stations of the workout more or less intense. To overload a circuit class, you may

1. Increase the number of stations.
2. Increase the number of repetitions performed at each station by increasing the duration or pace.
3. Repeat the number of times the circuit is repeated.
4. Increase the amount of weight used.

Two examples of a circuit workout are outlined in the "Circuit Routines" box. Circuit One alternates between step and body toning stations. Circuit Two interchanges floor aerobics with body toning stations. Use weights where it is applicable, and remember to go quickly from one station to the next. Do as many repetitions as the time will allow, but do not sacrifice technique for speed!

Cross-Training

Cross-training provides diversity in workout programs by including a variety of activities in a weekly workout routine. Cross-training programs allow for more individualized workout schedules and can maximize exercise benefits in a minimum amount of time. Activities include aerobics, anaerobics, strength, and flexibility exercises, as well as use of exercise machines to achieve training benefits. Fitness professionals claim that it is not difficult convincing exercise

CIRCUIT ROUTINES

	Circuit One (Step with Conditioning)	Circuit Two (Aerobics with Conditioning)
Station 1	Straddle step	Jumping jacks
Station 2	Squats with upright row	Squat with lateral raise
Station 3	Over the top with a double step	Jog in place
Station 4	Squats into a leg curl with shoulder press	Lunge with biceps curl
Station 5	Across the top with a double step	Alternate knee lift into jack
Station 6	Forward lunges with biceps curls	Push-up
Station 7	L step right and left	Jumping rope in place
Station 8	Stationary back lunges with lateral raises	Squat with side leg lift and shoulder press
Station 9	Repeater knees, side leg and back extension	Clap over and under leg
Station 10	Push-ups	Traveling lunges with biceps curl
Station 11	T step into power T step	Cha-chas forward and backward
Station 12	Abdominal curls	Abdominal curls

clients that cross-training is important to overall fitness improvement. Cross-training programs advocate that the student learn the basic principles of fitness, applying the overload principle to the exercise workouts to continually challenge muscle groups, and the specificity principle to not only develop areas of interest but also exercise new muscle groups to reach peak performance. Participants are also taught injury prevention, avoidance of overuse injuries, and diversity as a means of preventing exercise burnout. Cross-training allows participants to choose activities that they enjoy but also encourages them to try new activities. A typical weekly workout may include one day that combines an aerobic exercise class with 30 minutes on the weight machines, swimming or using the treadmill the next workout day, and aerobics and racquetball on the final workout day.

Cross-training has many benefits. Besides helping to increase awareness of total fitness, it

- Reduces injury due to overuse
- Provides a balance between cardiorespiratory training and strength training or muscular endurance training
- Promotes exercise modalities that increase coordination and flexibility
- Improves participants' adherence to exercise programs by adding variety

SUMMARY

Develop diversity in your workout schedule by trying the new and different types of aerobics classes described in this chapter, or by spicing up your workout with interval or circuit training. Develop your own weekly cross-training workout using your aerobics class as your basic activity, then adding one of the other types of aerobics classes described. Besides what we have discussed, don't forget some of the longtime standard aerobic activities: walking, jogging, running, rowing, cycling (road and mountain biking), swimming, and cross-country skiing. Use the personal fitness log at the end of this book (p. W-23) to record your additional aerobic activities performed outside of class. With such a great variety of activities available to promote total body fitness, there's really no excuse not to Keep Moving!

APPENDIX A

History of Aerobic Exercise

The concept of aerobic exercise is relatively new compared to the traditional methods of fitness, which premise that fitness is achieved through calisthenic exercise, weight training, or participation in sports. The fitness boom of the 1970s was preempted by Dr. Kenneth Cooper's research, which developed the concept of aerobic, or cardiorespiratory endurance training. Cooper's research on U.S. Air Force personnel determined that the key to aerobic fitness was the effectiveness of an individual's ability to take in and deliver oxygen to the body during exercise. Cooper concluded that the effectiveness of this ability, termed *oxygen consumption*, was the best way to determine an individual's fitness level.

Following his research, Cooper wrote a book entitled *Aerobics* (1968), which outlined his concept of aerobic exercise programs using traditional forms of exercise such as walking, jogging, swimming, and cycling. Cooper's exercise program used a point system whereby a person would work from their beginning fitness level and gradually progress toward a new fitness goal. Each exercise bout would carry a specific number of points determined by (1) the time it took, (2) the distance that was covered, (3) the frequency with which the exercise was performed. This set of performance guidelines was the beginning of the principles of fitness used today: *duration, intensity,* and *frequency.*

Cooper expanded his research and continued to publish additional fitness findings in his books *The New Aerobics* (1970) and *Aerobics for Women* (1972). The results of his publications helped to develop Americans' interest in fitness; what some people thought of as a fad became a historically significant national trend.

During this same time, Jacki Sorensen, while stationed at an Air Force Base in Puerto Rico with her husband, was asked to host a television exercise program for the base. While preparing for the show, she studied Cooper's Air Force Aerobics Program and participated in his 12-minute walk/run test. Sorensen scored "excellent" on the test and attributed her performance to the rigors of her years of dance training. In preparing for her TV broadcast, she combined Cooper's aerobic concepts with dance movements set to music to make the exercise fun and sociable. Sorensen's aerobic dance method appealed to people who did not like the more conventional modes of exercise and became widely popular particularly among women. After her return to the United States in 1971, Sorensen began to teach more aerobic dance classes. Eventually, she developed her own business franchise, Aerobic Dancing, Inc., and now has programs all across the United States, as well as in a few foreign countries. The results of her efforts have led aerobic dance aficionados to credit Jacki Sorensen as the founder of aerobic dance.

Another pioneer in aerobic dance history is Judi Sheppard Missett, the founder of Jazzercise, Inc. Like Sorensen, Judi Sheppard Missett originally began her career in dance. When Missett was teaching jazz dance, many of her women students were coming to class looking more for fitness training than for the technical training of dance. Missett revised her classes by creating simple dance routines that her students could follow without explanation and that sustained activity for the duration of the class. These changes increased the popularity of her classes and laid the foundations of her exercise program, Jazzercise. Today, Jazzercise is a thriving franchise business based solidly in jazz dance with a class structure typical of an aerobic dance class.

In the 1980s, with aerobics no longer in its infancy, participants and instructors alike sought new and creative ways to make aerobics classes more fun and challenging. New and various forms of aerobic exercise classes were introduced in the hope they would please the public and motivate participants to continue in fitness training. In the late 1980s, Gin Miller, a former gymnast, developed step aerobics. Miller had been using bench-stepping equipment for rehabilitation and therapeutic purposes. As she worked with the step bench, she realized the endless choreographic possibilities within this piece of equipment. Step aerobics has created a great deal of enthusiasm and is as popular a form of aerobics as is aerobic dance.

Aerobics has become recognized by fitness experts as a means to good health. In the 1980s, the American College of Sports Medicine determined that three aerobic workouts a week were necessary for the maintenance of cardiorespiratory fitness. The media has responded to the public's quest for fitness with television exercise shows and videos to satisfy all fitness levels. Floor aerobics and step aerobics provide the foundations for aerobic workout classes while new innovations in aerobic fitness continue to find their way into the aerobic studio. Slide aerobics, cardiofunk, Yogaerobics, and jump rope training are providing aerobic exercisers with other workout options. Water fitness classes are making a big splash, while boxing and martial-arts-based aerobic programs are punching and kicking their way into the aerobic limelight. Group indoor cycling is an activity that appeals to men and women alike as they pedal up and down imaginary roads to fitness.

Dr. Kenneth Cooper's research began the aerobics craze. Aerobic exercise continues to grow in popularity as many new and exciting changes continue to emerge. The history of aerobics today is brief, but it is just the beginning!

APPENDIX B

A Career in Fitness

The available opportunities for a career in fitness have been limited until recent years. Traditionally, for individuals interested in a career in fitness, the primary career choice has been in the educational field. Today, however, the field of fitness offers career opportunities not only in education but in health centers, fitness facilities, and as independent contractors working as fitness trainers. Although a college degree is certainly a calling card for a job interview, many certificated programs offer training background in preparedness for employment as a fitness instructor.

To begin a career as an aerobics instructor, you can enroll in a training course that will teach the skills needed to be a safe and effective aerobics teacher. National organizations host certificate programs, primarily on a weekend basis. Community colleges and university continuing education programs offer courses that are more in-depth, presenting and reviewing material over the course of several weeks or for a full quarter or semester. With successful completion of one of these training courses, you can obtain the certificate required for becoming an aerobics instructor.

All nationally recognized examination programs have a required curriculum that includes information regarding training principles standard to the industry. Before enrolling for a national certification examination, it would be best to study courses that provide background knowledge for the exam. These courses should include a general knowledge of exercise science, anatomy and kinesiology, nutrition, and sports injuries and rehabilitation. Skills in aerobic

movement, choreography, and appropriate teaching techniques should also be incorporated into preparation for the certification. Student teaching experience would help develop experience as a group exercise leader.

In seeking employment, there are a variety of organizations and private businesses that offer exercise programs. Aerobics classes can be taught at health and fitness clubs, recreation centers, schools, senior centers, hospitals, corporations, churches—the list is almost endless!

As a fitness instructor, you may also want to become involved in a career as a personal trainer. Like aerobics instructors, personal trainers must also pass certifying exams. Background study for these exams would be similar to that suggested for studies in aerobic certification with the addition of an in-depth knowledge of weight-lifting skills and techniques. Personal trainers should have abilities to develop individualized workout programs based on the client's desire to develop particular areas of fitness, or to serve as a supplement training program for sports competition. As a personal trainer, having skill in time management is essential to developing a business that can accommodate the scheduling needs of a variety of clients. Because personal trainers may work privately as well as for a fitness organization, it is essential to investigate the liability responsibilities of this profession.

In the expanding field of fitness, various other career opportunities are available. Supervisory or management positions in recreational programs or at fitness facilities; research in fitness, athletic training, dance therapy; or exercise rehabilitation are a few of the possible career opportunities now available in the fitness industry. However, these careers generally require more than a certification, and most often a college or university degree is the minimum qualification for job application. Luckily, the way to a career in fitness is no longer along a single path. Career opportunities are increasing for individuals who love movement and exercise and who want to share the joy of fitness.

APPENDIX C

Exercise Recommendations for Special Populations

PREGNANT WOMEN

Many women ask if they should continue doing aerobics when they become pregnant. The answer to this question depends on many issues. If someone is already involved in an aerobics program and they are in good health, if the pregnancy has no risks, and if the woman's physician gives consent, then it is to the woman's advantage to continue exercising.

However, if the woman has never been involved in an exercise program, consent from the doctor is necessary before proceeding in exercise activity. Exercise choices should be low intensity and low impact, such as walking, swimming, stationary bicycling, or other nonimpact activities. If pregnant women choose to embark on an aerobics program, they should attend a prenatal aerobics class. Such classes have become popular and are offered through recreation departments, YMCAs, YWCAs, and other community centers.

Exercise Guidelines

Whether you are exercising in a group setting or individually, there are specific guidelines that have been defined by the American College of Obstetricians and Gynecologists (ACOG) that are important for prenatal and postnatal care. The ACOG guidelines are based on the unique physiological conditions that exist during pregnancy and the postpartum period. These criteria should provide direction to prenatal and post-partum patients during their participation in exercise programs. Your obstetrician should have a detailed outline of these (ACOG) guidelines, or you may write directly to the organization in Washington, D.C.

As they relate to the concept of aerobics that we have defined in this book, the ACOG guidelines specify the following general exercise parameters.

Recommendations for Exercise in Pregnancy and Postpartum

There are no data in humans to indicate that pregnant women should limit exercise intensity and lower target heart rates because of potential adverse effects. For women who do not have any additional risk factors for adverse maternal or perinatal outcome, the following recommendations may be made:

1. During pregnancy, women can continue to exercise and derive health benefits even from mild-to-moderate exercise routines. Regular exercise (at least three times per week) is preferable to intermittent activity.

2. Women should avoid exercise in the supine position after the first trimester. Such a position is associated with decreased cardiac output in most pregnant women; because the remaining cardiac output will be preferentially distributed away from splanchnic beds (including the uterus) during vigorous exercise, such regimens are best avoided

during pregnancy. Prolonged periods of motionless standing should also be avoided.

3. Women should be aware of the decreased oxygen available for aerobic exercise during pregnancy. They should be encouraged to modify the intensity of their exercise according to maternal symptoms. Pregnant women should stop exercising when fatigued and not exercise to exhaustion. Weight-bearing exercises may under some circumstances be continued at intensities similar to those prior to pregnancy throughout pregnancy. Non-weight-bearing exercises such as cycling or swimming will minimize the risk of injury and facilitate the continuation of exercise during pregnancy.

4. Morphologic changes in pregnancy should serve as a relative contraindication to types of exercise in which loss of balance could be detrimental to maternal or fetal well-being, especially in the third trimester. Further, any type of exercise involving the potential for even mild abdominal trauma should be avoided.

5. Pregnancy requires an additional 300 kcal/d in order to maintain metabolic homeostasis. Thus, women who exercise during pregnancy should be particularly careful to ensure an adequate diet.

6. Pregnant women who exercise in the first trimester should augment heat dissipation by ensuring adequate hydration, appropriate clothing, and optimal environmental surroundings during exercise.

7. Many of the physiologic and morphologic changes of pregnancy persist 4 to 6 weeks postpartum. Thus, prepregnancy exercise routines should be resumed gradually based on a woman's physical capability.

It is important to be especially aware of how you are feeling when you are exercising. Unlike fitness levels when you are not pregnant, as you progress in pregnancy, you must decrease the intensity of the exercise and instead of applying overload, the load must be lightened.

Exercising when pregnant can be a very positive experience. If you follow safe guidelines and recommendations, it will help ease the pregnancy and postpartum process. Being in good physical condition can promote a quicker recovery but, unfortunately, cannot guarantee an easy labor.

With your physician's approval, continue or renew your exercise program. Find the activity that suits your needs, and make sure to stay within the recommended guidelines for a safe and healthy pregnancy!

OLDER ADULTS

Perhaps we should consider exercise to be our fountain of youth. Although the aging process is inevitable, exercise has been shown to be able to reduce the effects of aging, and even postpone some of the physiological changes that occur with aging. As we age, modifications to exercise should accommodate the changes.

There are normal physiological changes that occur with aging:

Maximum heart rate declines.

Maximal oxygen uptake declines.

Bones become more fragile. Osteoporosis (a gradual loss or thinning of the bone) is a major concern of the elderly.

Skeletal muscle mass declines, resulting in a loss of muscular strength and endurance.

Connective tissue becomes stiffer and joints become less mobile. Loss of flexibility may be the result of the underlying degenerative disease called arthritis (a stiffening of the joints).

Lean body weight declines and body fat increases.

Basal metabolic rate declines.

Resting heart rate increases.

Exercise can affect these normal changes.

Exercise Guidelines

As an older adult, when you exercise, and if you choose aerobics as your exercise, make sure to follow these guidelines for a safe and effective workout.

1. Before starting an exercise program, consult a physician.
2. Follow these exercise parameters:
   - *Frequency.*—3 to 4 times a week.
   - *Duration.*—A minimum of 20 minutes
   - *Intensity.*—60 to 70 percent of maximum heart rate
3. Do not exercise in the extreme heat and humidity.
4. Use layered clothing to prevent overheating or cooling. Older adults are less tolerant of the heat and cold.
5. Warm up thoroughly, and then gradually increase the intensity from a low to moderate pace.
6. Avoid fast transitions to prevent dizziness or falling.
7. Limit the number of repetitions of an exercise, especially those involving the knee and shoulder joint. Overuse is a common injury to the older adult.
8. Drink plenty of liquids throughout the exercise session to rehydrate the body.
9. Monitor exercise intensity frequently.
10. If you are on medication, special precautions should be taken and consistent medical consultation is recommended.
11. An extended cool-down is encouraged as a means to enhance flexibility and prevent muscle soreness.

By the year 2030, it is estimated that 20 percent of the population will be over 65. With these statistics, it is important that the population maintains good health. With good exercise habits, this 20 percent of the population will not only have an extended life span, but they will be able to enjoy their life in good health!

OBESE PERSONS

The problem of obesity, defined by the American College of Sports Medicine as body fat levels for women that exceed 30 percent and for men, 25 percent, is not necessarily merely the result of overeating. A wide variety of influences may contribute to the excessive weight gain: eating habits, environment, social factors, body image, and biochemical differences that can affect resting metabolic rate. The treatment procedures for obesity in the past—diets, drugs, psychological treatment, group weight-loss programs, surgery, exercise programs—have often failed to resolve the problem on a long-term basis.

Another definition of obesity refers to the size and number of fat cells. Each individual fat cell can enlarge (hypertrophy), and the total number of fat cells can increase (hyperplasia). An increase in the number of fat cells can occur at three life periods: the first year of life, the growth-spurt period of adolescence, and the last trimester of pregnancy. Because the number of fat cells becomes stable sometime before adulthood, any weight gain or loss after that time is related to a change in the size of the fat cells.

Obesity often begins in childhood. If a child is overfat, it is not unlikely that fatness will continue through adulthood. Excessive fatness can also develop slowly during the adult ages of 25 to 44. Differences exist in risks due to obesity in Black adult males as compared to white men. There is also an increased chance of obesity in women as compared to men in the age range of 25 to 34.

Obesity can cause health problems such as high blood pressure, heart disease, and arthritis, and is associated with diabetes. Obesity can increase the risk of gallbladder disease, increase risk during surgery, and may decrease life expectancy. However, regular exercise throughout life controls excess weight gain. Increases in body fat seem to be more a result of lack of activity than overeating or age.

For people who are overweight, engaging in a regular exercise regime tends to decrease their food intake, despite the additional caloric output of exercise activity. Body fat decreases and, with continued regular exercise, lean body mass increases. There is also an increase in the basal metabolic rate, which brings about changes in enzymes that facilitate fat metabolism in the tissues. Eventually, a regular exercise routine helps to balance food intake and energy requirements so that a new lower level of body mass is attained.

To achieve a successful fitness exercise program for someone who is obese, the emphasis should be on *exercise frequency* and *duration*. In an obese person, excess weight places greater demands on the musculoskeletal system, thus making the stress placed on connective tissue and joints more of a risk factor. Also, cardiovascular demands are greater in an obese person. As a result of these risk factors, the intensity of the exercise program should be low. Lower intensity offers less physical trauma. The obese person need only exercise in the target training zone for approximately 5 to 10 minutes

as compared to a minimum of 20 minutes for a person of normal weight. (As the obese person loses weight, this time length will gradually increase as fitness increases.) Because the length of time or duration of activity is short, the frequency of the exercise program should be 5 to 6 days per week. A sound fitness program should include an exercise mode that will offer a person maximum caloric expenditure. Water aerobics is an excellent exercise program choice, as is a walking program. Low-impact aerobics is considered a good selection once a person has increased the length of time they are able to exercise in the target training zone to 15 to 20 minutes. Step aerobics is not recommended because of the high intensity of this fitness program.

It is recommended that a person who is obese obtain a health care professional's approval before engaging in an exercise program. Once recommendations have been obtained, it is important to establish a safe, regular exercise program as a *lifetime* commitment.

APPENDIX D

Music and Video Resources

Any music store will have a wide variety of aerobic music. The choice depends on what appeals to you. Rhythmic and upbeat music is most appropriate for much of the class; however, the flexibility cool-down segment is best suited to slow, mellow music that encourages relaxation. Besides music stores, there are many companies nationwide that make audio tapes and compact discs specifically for aerobics classes. Following is a list of companies that provide this service:

1. Power Music
   1303 Swaner Rd.
   Salt Lake City, UT 84104
   1-800-777-Beat
   Fax: 801-975-7774
   E-mail: workout@powermusic.com

2. Dancetracks!
   AE1 Music Network, Inc.
   72 Spring St., Suite 1004
   New York, NY 10012
   1-800-AE1-MUSIC

3. Muscle Mixes Music
   P.O. Box 533967
   Orlando, FL 32853-3967
   1-800-52-Mixes
   Fax: 407-872-7582
   E-mail: Sonja@musclemixes.com

4. Pacesetter Music
   P.O. Box 57
   5472 S. 7100 W.
   Hooper, UT 84315-0057
   801-773-2000

5. Musicflex Inc.
   159-34 90th St.
   Queens, NY 11414
   718-738-MUFX or
   1-800-430-3539
   Fax: 718-843-6598

6. Mix Music International Inc.
   P.O. Box 2452
   Kankakee, IL 60901
   1-800-733-3049

7. Ken Alan Associates
   7985 Santa Monica Blvd., #109
   Los Angeles, CA 90046
   1-800-KEN-6060

8. Dynamix
   733 W. 40th St.
   Suite 10
   Baltimore, MD 21211
   1-800-843-6499
   Fax: 410-243-9759
   E-mail: dynamix@dynamix-music.com

9. PROmotion Music
   1611 N. Stemmons Fwy., #416
   Carrollton, TX 75006
   1-800-380-4776
   Fax: 972-446-3144
   E-mail: comments@promotionmusic.com

If you are building a fitness library, or merely want to rent a video for a home workout, you will want to select a video that includes a well-rounded workout program, with sound instructional techniques and safety standards. Consider the following criteria for evaluating a video:

Does the workout include an adequate warm-up and cool-down stretch?

Is the workout appropriate for your participation level, or are there a variety of levels to select from?

Does the instructor provide heart rate checks during the aerobic activity?

Does the instructor perform movements using proper technique?

Is there clear cueing for movements by the instructor?

Does the tape have good audiovisual quality with easy-to-follow camera angles?

Does the workout include exercises for opposing muscle groups?

Does the instructor include safety precautions for exercises?

Is the overall presentation and workout motivational?

Because new exercise videos are continually entering the marketplace, you may want to send away for a catalog that is always updated and does a careful screening of any videotape they have included. This catalog, entitled *The Complete Guide to Exercise Videos,* can be received for a nominal fee by writing to

Collage Video Specialities Inc.
5390 Main Street NE, Dept. 1
Minneapolis, MN 55421

or by calling the toll-free number

1-800-433-6769
Fax: 612-571-5906
E-mail: collage@collagevideo.com

The catalog contains the names of the best exercise videos available, with a detailed explanation of each tape. They will mail order any videotape listed in their catalog. They also supply audio tapes appropriate for aerobics.

APPENDIX E

Suggested Reading List

AEROBICS AND FITNESS

Bailey, Covert. *Fit or Fat.* Boston: Houghton Mifflin, 1978.

——. *The New Fit or Fat.* Boston: Houghton Mifflin, 1991.

Bailey, Covert, and Lea Bishop. *The Fit or Fat Woman.* Boston: Houghton Mifflin, 1989.

Brooks, George A., Thomas D. Fahey, and Timothy P. White. *Exercise Physiology: Human Bioenergetics and Its Applications,* 2nd ed. Mountain View, CA: Mayfield, 1996.

Cooper, Kenneth H. *Aerobics for Women.* New York: Bantam, 1980.

——. *The Aerobics Program for Total Well-Being.* New York: Bantam, 1983.

Cooper, Phyllis Gorney, ed. *Aerobics: Theory and Practice.* Costa Mesa, CA: HDL Publishing, 1988.

Cotton, Richard T. *Aerobics Instructor Manual.* San Diego, CA: American Council on Exercise, 1993.

Donovan, Grant, Jane McNamara, and Peter Gianoli. *Exercise Danger.* Dubuque, IA: Kendall/Hunt, 1988.

Fahey, T. D., P. M. Insel, and W. T. Roth. *Fit & Well,* 3rd ed. Mountain View, CA: Mayfield, 1999.

Fitness Magazine, G and J USA Publishing Co., 2 West 45th St., New York, NY 10006.

Fox, Edward, Timothy Kirby, and Ann Roberts Fox. *Bases of Fitness.* New York: Macmillan, 1987.

Gelder, Naneene Van. *Aerobic Dance-Exercise Instructor Manual.* San Diego: IDEA Foundation, 1987.

Kravitz, Len. *Anybody's Guide to Total Fitness.* Dubuque, IA: Kendall/Hunt, 1989.

McIntosh, Mathew. *Lifetime Aerobics.* Dubuque, IA: William C. Brown, 1990.

Shape Magazine, Shape Magazine Inc., 21100 Erwin St., Woodland Hills, CA 91367.

Thaxton, Nolan. *Pathways to Fitness.* New York: Harper and Row, 1988.

Woman's Sports and Fitness, Woman's Sports and Fitness Inc., 2025 Pearl St., Boulder, CO 80302.

FLEXIBILITY

Alter, Micheal J. *Sport Stretch.* Champaign, IL: Leisure Press, 1990.

——. *Science of Stretching.* Champaign, IL: Human Kinetics Books, 1988.

——. *Science of Flexibility,* 2nd ed. Champaign, IL: Human Kinetics Publishers, 1996.

Martins, Peter. *The New York City Ballet Workout: Fifty Stretches and Exercises Anyone Can Do for a Strong, Graceful, and Sculpted Body.* New York: William Morrow, 1997.

McAtee, Robert E. *Facilitated Stretching.* Champaign, IL: Human Kinetics Publishers, 1993.

Smith, Bob. *Flexibility for Sport.* Wiltshire, Eng.: Crowood Press, 1997.

St. George, Francine. *Stretching for Flexibility and Health*. Freedom, CA: Crossing Press, 1997.

INJURIES

Arnheim, Daniel D. *Modern Principles of Athletic Training*, 7th ed. St. Louis: Times Mirror/ Mosby, 1985.

Fahey, Tom. *Athletic Training: Principles and Practice*. Palo Alto, CA: Mayfield, 1986.

Guten, Gary N. *Play Healthy, Stay Healthy*. Champaign, IL: Leisure Press, 1991.

Morris, Alfred. *Sports Medicine: Prevention of Athletic Injuries*. Dubuque, IA: Brown, 1984.

Ritter, M. A., and M. J. Albohm. *Your Injury: A Commonsense Guide to the Management of Sports Injury*. Indianapolis: Benchmark, 1987.

Solomon, Ruth, Sandra Minton, and John Solomon. *Preventing Dance Injuries*. Waldorf, MD: American Alliance, 1990.

NUTRITION

Bailey, Covert. *Fit or Fit Target Diet*. Boston: Houghton Mifflin, 1994.

Brody, Jane. *Jane Brody's Good Food Book: Living the High Carbohydrate Way*. New York: W. W. Norton, 1985.

Burke, L. "Practical Issues in Nutrition for Athletes." *Journal of Sports Sciences* 13 (Spec.) S80–S83, 1995.

Clark, Nancy. *The Athlete's Kitchen*. New York: Bantam, 1983.

——. *Sports Nutrition Guidebook*. Champaign, IL: Leisure Press, 1990.

Coleman, Ellen. *Eating for Endurance*. Palo Alto, CA: Bull Publishing, 1988.

Coleman, Ellen, and Susan Nelson Steen. *The Ultimate Sports Nutrition Handbook*. Palo Alto, CA: Bull Publishing, 1996.

Dusky, Lorraine, and J. J. Leedy. *How to Eat Like a Thin Person*. New York: Simon and Schuster, 1982.

Franz, Marion J. *Fast Food Facts*. Minneapolis: International Diabetes Center, 1987.

Nieman, David C. *Exercise Testing and Prescription: A Health-Related Approach*, 4th ed. Mountain View, CA: Mayfield, 1999.

Tribole, Evelyn. *Eating on the Run*. Champaign, IL: Leisure Press, 1992.

APPENDIX F

Exercise Websites

Internet Fitness Resource
http://www.netsweat.com/
Start here. Every link an aerobics student on the Internet could wish for. Absolutely amazing.

Spinning on the net
http://www.spinning.com
The official Internet site for Spinning.

SoBe Fit
http://www.sobefit.com/welcome.htm
The website includes a music library for aerobics courses and competitive aerobics, an archive of and forum for exchanging choreographic ideas, and relevant articles.

AFAA TeleFitness Center
http://www.aerobics.com/10000.asp?1=
The latest information on staying in shape, *Fitness Magazine* on-line, and fitness triage, where you can find out what your exercise risks are through a program that evaluates your fitness level and risks.

TurnStep
http://www.turnstep.com/
A library of aerobics patterns with graphics; you can use it to start working on your own choreography.

MiningCo Exercise page
http://www.exercise.miningco.com/mbody.htm?COB=home&PID=2756
A great resource for links to other fitness sites.

Video fitness — consumer guide
http://www.videofitness.com/
Trying to pick out an exercise video? Here's a consumer's guide to fitness videos.

Fitness Online magazine
http://www.fitnessonline.com
Along with a database of workouts, and a health calculator, this site includes the on-line versions of a number of fitness magazines including *Shape, Flex,* and *Living Fit.*

StayInShape
http://www.stayinshape.com
Includes a nutritional database that gives you information on edibles, as well as relevant articles and a fitness directory to help you find a gym.

GLOSSARY

aerobic Literally means "with oxygen." Aerobic exercise utilizes oxygen in order to recycle ATP and in turn contract the working muscle.

agonist muscle The muscle group that is the prime mover of contraction in an exercise.

alignment The relationship of the body segments to one another.

anaerobic Literally means "without oxygen." Anaerobic exercise recycles ATP and in turn contracts the working muscle without utilizing oxygen.

anaerobic glycolysis The energy system that uses only the stored glycogen in our muscle cells to resynthesize ATP. This energy system is used for intense bursts of energy and lasts for only the first 2 minutes of exercise.

antagonist muscle The muscle group that opposes the prime mover (agonist) muscle. The antagonist muscle is usually stretched while the prime mover is contracted.

arrhythmia Abnormal heartbeat.

ATP (adenosine triphosphate) A substance that must be present in the muscle cell in order for the muscle to contract.

ballistic stretch A stretch that uses body momentum to force the muscle groups into as much extensibility as can be tolerated.

BMR (basal metabolic rate) The energy output to maintain life functions—respiration, digestion, circulation and nerve, hormonal, and cellular activities.

body composition The total of fat weight and lean body weight. The assessment of body composition determines the body's percentages of fat and lean weight.

calorie The unit of measure that indicates the amount of energy released by food.

cardiac output The total amount of blood the heart pumps in one minute.

cardiorespiratory endurance The ability of the cardiovascular system (heart and blood vessels) and the respiratory system (lungs and air passages) to function efficiently during sustained, vigorous activities (also called *cardiovascular endurance*).

circuit training A specific exercise or routine that is performed in a given period of time. Once completed, a new exercise or routine is performed with a specific time frame. A series of these timed exercises is called a *circuit*.

complex carbohydrates One of the two types of carbohydrates, which supply the body with its primary source of energy, glucose. Complex carbohydrates are starches, and include the natural sugars found in fruits, vegetables, and grains. *See also* simple carbohydrates.

concentric contraction The phase of the isotonic muscular contraction in which the muscle shortens.

creatine phosphate A phosphagen, similar to ATP, that is stored in the muscle cells and used as an immediate energy source for anaerobic activity.

cross-training A type of training program that includes a variety of activities in a weekly workout routine.

diastolic blood pressure A measure of the resting pressure in the arteries when the heart is not contracting.

eccentric contraction   The phase of isotonic muscular contraction in which the muscle lengthens.

endurance   The ability of a muscle or group of muscles to perform work (repeated muscular contractions) for a long time.

flexibility   The range of motion of a certain joint and its corresponding muscle groups.

glycogen   The storage form of glucose. It is found in large amounts in the muscle cells and the liver. It serves as an important source of energy during exercise.

hemoglobin   A protein cell present in the blood that transports oxygen to the working muscle.

interval training   Series of high-intensity exercises alternated with periods of rest.

isometric contraction   A muscle contraction that produces force without changing the length of the muscle.

isotonic contraction   A shortening of concentric muscle contraction that creates movement.

kilocalorie   The energy food releases, measured in calories.

kyphosis   A postural deviation where the muscles of the upper back are weakened and therefore develop a rounded or hunched appearance.

lactic acid   The end product of anaerobic glycolysis. As lactic acid builds in a muscle cell, the muscle fatigues and muscular contraction becomes increasingly difficult.

lipid   Any of a group of organic compounds consisting of the fats and other substances of similar properties.

lordosis   An extreme forward tilt of the pelvic girdle. In this position, the abdominal muscles are overstretched and the lower back muscles are overcontracted (also called *swayback*).

metabolism   The body's process of converting food into energy through numerous chemical reactions.

muscular endurance   The ability of local skeletal muscles to perform work strenuously for progressively longer periods of time.

overload principle   The ability of the body to adapt to higher performance levels and gradually increase its capacity to do more work.

perceived exertion   A self-test used during the aerobic workout to detect signs of fatigue. The perceived exertion scale was formalized by Borg in 1982.

phosphagen energy system   The energy system named after the presence of creatine phosphate, which exists in the muscle cells. The phosphagen energy system is utilized in the initial burst of energy for muscular contraction.

phospholipid   One of the three types of lipids found in food; a combination of one or more fatty acid molecules with phosphoric acid and a nitrogen base. *See also* lipid, sterol, triglyceride.

placement   The relative positioning of the individual body parts.

posture   The position of the body as it is held in space.

progression   A gradual increase in the overload of a workout. Progression can be applied to the duration, intensity, or frequency of the workout.

recovery heart rate   The heart rate 1 minute after exercise is stopped, which indicates how quickly you recover from exercise.

resting heart rate   The heart rate taken just after waking up in the morning.

scoliosis   A deformity in which the spine is bent to one side.

simple carbohydrates   One of the two types of carbohydrates, which supply the body with its primary source of energy, glucose. Simple carbohydrates are sugars, and include maltose (found in malt), lactose (in milk), and sucrose (in table sugar). *See also* complex carbohydrates.

slide aerobics   A type of training program in which a lateral movement trainer is used to perform aerobic conditioning movements and exercises.

somatotype   A system for classifying the three general body types: endomorph, mesomorph, and ectomorph.

specificity principle The ability of the body to adapt specifically to the demands placed on it.

static stretch A position of extreme stretch on a given muscle group that is assumed and held for a period of time.

step workout A type of aerobic conditioning that uses a low bench to perform specific exercises.

sterol One of three types of lipids found in food; cholesterol is the most widely known sterol. *See also* lipid, sterol, triglyceride.

strength The ability of a muscle or group of muscles to exert a force against a resistance in one all-out effort.

stroke volume The amount of blood the heart pumps per beat.

synergist muscle The muscle group that assists but is not the prime mover (agonist) in an exercise.

systolic blood pressure A measure of the rhythmic contraction of the heart as blood leaves it through the ventricles. Systolic blood pressure rises with increased cardiac output.

talk test A method for measuring the intensity of an aerobic activity. You must be able to carry on a conversation during exercise, or the intensity of the activity is too great.

target heart rate The rate at which your heart must work in order to affect your aerobic capacity (also called the *exercise heart rate*).

tempo The speed at which a piece of music is performed.

threshold of training The minimum amount of exercise necessary to produce improvements in physical fitness.

training effect The physiological changes that occur in the body due to regular and proper participation in a fitness program.

triglyceride One of the three types of lipids found in food; triglycerides make up approximately 98 percent of our fat intake from food. *See also* lipid, phospholipid, sterol.

REFERENCES

1. Allsen, Philip E. *Conditioning and Physical Fitness*. Dubuque, IA: Brown, 1978.

2. American College of Obstetricians and Gynecologists. *Exercise During Pregnancy and Postnatal Period*. Washington, DC: ACOG, 1985.

3. American College of Sports Medicine. "Recommendations and Quality of Exercise for Developing and Maintaining Fitness in Healthy Adults." *Journal of Physical Education and Recreation* 51, no. 5 (May 1980): 17–18.

4. American Council on Exercise. *Aerobics Instructor Manual*. San Diego, 1993.

5. Astrand, P., and K. Rodahl. *Textbook of Work Physiology*. New York: McGraw Hill, 1977.

6. Bailey, Covert. *Fit or Fat?* Boston: Houghton Mifflin, 1977.

7. Bucher, Charles A., and William E. Prentice. *Fitness for College and Life*. St. Louis: Times/Mirror, Mosby, 1985.

8. Cantu, Robert C. *Clinical Sports Medicine*. Lexington, MA: Heath, 1983.

9. Corbin, Charles B., and Ruth Lindsey. *Concepts of Fitness*. Dubuque, IA: Brown, 1985.

10. Day, Nancy Raines. "Footowner's Manual: A Guide to Good Foot Care." *Shape Magazine* (July 1985).

11. DeVries, H. A. *Physiology of Exercise for Physical Education and Athletics*, 3d ed. Dubuque, IA: Brown, 1980.

12. Dintiman, George B., Stephen E. Stone, Jude C. Pennington, and Robert G. Davis. *Discovering Lifetime Fitness: Concepts of Exercise and Weight Control*. St. Paul, MN: West, 1984.

13. Dowdy, Deborah, Kirk J. Cureton, Harry P. DuVal, and Harvey G. Outz. "Effects of Aerobic Dance on Physical Work Capacity, Cardiovascular Function, and Body Composition of Middle-aged Women. *Research Quarterly for Exercise and Sport* 56, no. 3 (1985): 227–233.

14. Fahey, Thomas D. *Athletic Training: Principles and Practices*. Mountain View, CA: Mayfield, 1986.

15. Fahey, Thomas D., Paul M. Insel, and Walton T. Roth. *Fit & Well,* 3rd ed. Mountain View, CA: Mayfield, 1999.

16. Falls, Harold B., Ann M. Baylor, and Rod K. Dishman. *Essentials of Fitness*. Philadelphia: SCP, 1980.

17. Fleck, Steven J., and William J. Kraemer. "The Overtraining Syndrome." *NSCA Journal* (August, September 1982).

18. Fox, Edward L., Richard W. Bowers, and Merle L. Foss. *The Physiological Basis of Physical Education and Athletics*. Philadelphia: Saunders, 1988.

19. Fox, S. M., J. P. Naughton, and W. L. Hackell. "Physical Activity: The Prevention of Coronary Heart Disease." *Annals of Clinical Research* 3 (1971): 404–432.

20. Francis, Kennon T. "Delayed Muscle Soreness: A Review." *Journal of Orthopedic and Sports Physical Therapy* (1983).

21. Francis, Lorna L. *Injury Prevention Manual for Dance Exercises*. San Diego: National Injury Prevention Foundation, 1983.

22. Gelder, Naneene Van, ed. *Aerobic Dance — Exercise Instructor Manual*. San Diego: IDEA Foundation, 1987.

23. Getchell, Bud. *Physical Fitness: A Way of Life,* 3d ed. New York: Macmillan, 1983.

24. Goodman Kraines, Minda, and Esther Kan. *Jump into Jazz*. Palo Alto, CA: Mayfield, 1983.

25. Hallander, Jane. "Cardiokickboxing Fitness for the Millenium." *Martial Arts Illustrated* (November 1998), pp. 46–51.

26. Jensen, Clayne R., and Garth A. Fisher. *Scientific Basis of Athletic Conditioning*, 2d ed. Philadelphia: Lea and Febiger, 1979.

27. Krepton, Dorie, and Donald Chu, *Everybody's Aerobic Book,* Edina, MN: Bellwether Press, 1986.

28. Lamb, David R. *Physiology of Exercise: Response and Adaptations,* 2d ed. New York: Macmillan, 1984.

29. McArdle, William D., Frank I. Katch, and Victor I. Katch. *Exercise Physiology: Energy, Nutrition, and Human Performance.* Philadelphia: Lea & Febiger, 1981.

30. Mylrea, Mindy. *1997 World Fitness IDEA Convention Guide.* IDEA, pp. 535–545, 1997.

31. Patton, John Pitchforth. "The Aerobic Kickboxing Craze; *Blackbelt* (December 1997), pp. 48–53.

32. Pollock, M. L., J. H. Wilmore, and S. M. Fox. *Exercise in Health and Disease.* Philadelphia: Saunders, 1984.

33. Rasch, P. J., and R. K. Burke. *Kinesiology and Applied Anatomy,* 6th ed. Philadelphia: Lea & Febiger, 1978.

34. Sharkey, Brian J. *Physiology of Fitness.* Champaign, IL: Human Kinetics, 1979.

35. Williams, Melvin. *Lifetime Physical Fitness.* Dubuque, IA: Brown, 1985.

WORKSHEETS

MEDICAL PROFILE

Name ——————————————————— Date ———————————————

Age ——————————— Days/Time Class Meets ——————————————

Local Address ———————————————————————————————

Business Phone ——————————— Home Phone ——————————————

SS Number ————————————————

Have you had previous instruction in aerobics? ——————————————————

If yes, where and for how long? —————————————————————————

Are you currently involved in a regular program of aerobics? ————————————

If yes, what type of aerobic activity? ————————————————————————

Please list reasons for taking this course and any personal goals you wish to achieve:

Please check in the appropriate space if you have any of these conditions and if they would limit your participation in class:

—— allergies   —— heart disease

—— arthritis   —— high blood pressure

—— asthma   —— pregnant*

—— diabetes   —— smoking

—— dysmenorrhea   —— migraine

—— epilepsy   —— other

Do you take any medication on a regular basis? ———————————————————

If so, indicate what type. ——————————————————————————————

Reason: ————————————————————————————————————

I am aware of my medical profile. I will proceed with my exercise program at a "safe" level.

SIGNATURE ——————————————— DATE ———————————————

* If you should become pregnant after the class term has begun, please inform the instructor so that your exercise can be modified appropriately. A physican's consent is encouraged for continued participation.

FITNESS PROFILE

NAME _____

INITIAL LEVEL	END-OF-SEMESTER LEVEL

HEART RATE

Resting _____   Resting _____

Target _____   Target _____

CARDIORESPIRATORY PERFORMANCE EXAMS

1.5-Run/3-Mile Walk Test

Time _____   Time _____

Fitness Level _____   Fitness Level _____

3-Minute Step Test

Heart Rate _____   Heart Rate _____

Fitness Level _____   Fitness Level _____

MUSCULAR STRENGTH AND ENDURANCE

Curl-up Test

Number _____   Number _____

Fitness Level _____   Fitness Level _____

Push-up Test

Number _____   Number _____

Fitness Level _____   Fitness Level _____

FLEXIBILITY

Self-Test Flexibility Evaluations

Enter pass or fail for each of the following:

Quadriceps   _____   _____

Calves
(gastrocnemius/soleus)   _____   _____

Lower back   _____   _____

Hip flexor
(iliopsoas)   _____   _____

Hamstrings   _____   _____

BODY COMPOSITION

_____ %   _____ %

Fitness Level _____   Fitness Level _____

GIRTH MEASUREMENTS

CHEST	Take from behind. Have another person place tape across nipple line.
ABDOMEN	Horizontal measures taken at the level of the umbilicus.
CALF	Measure the *maximum* circumference between the knee and ankle. Have person put foot on chair to measure.
FOREARM	With the arms slightly away from the trunk in anatomical position, take a perpendicular measure to the long axis of the forearm at the level of maximum circumference.
HIPS/BUTTOCKS	Horizontal measures at the maximum circumference of the hip/buttocks region. Measure at widest part of the buttocks.
ARM/BICEPS	Take at belly of muscle.
WAIST	Horizontal measure taken at the narrowest part of the torso.
HIPS/THIGHS	Horizontal measures taken at the maximum circumference of the hip/thighs just *below* the gluteal region.
THIGH	Horizontal measures taken at the top part of thigh at maximum circumference.

P R O C E D U R E S

✔ *Take measurements on the right side of the body.*

✔ *Pull tape to proper tension without pinching the skin.*

✔ *Take 2–3 measurements at each site.*

✔ *Retest if measurements do not fall within .25 inches or 7mm.*

Chest _____	Hips/Buttocks _____	Thigh (1) _____
Abdomen _____	Arm/Biceps _____	Waist/Hip Ratio _____
Calf _____	Waist _____	Rating: Women <0.8
Forearm _____	Hips/Thighs _____	Rating: Men <0.9

CALCULATING RESTING HEART RATE

Name _____ Class Day/Time _____

DIRECTIONS

Take your heart rate for 60 seconds, first thing in the morning before you get out of bed. Lightly press your first three fingers at either the radial (at the wrist) or carotid (side of the neck) artery. Record the number of beats counted. Repeat this procedure for 3 consecutive days and then take the average of the total.

PRETEST

DATE _____

Day 1 _____ BPM (beats per minute)

Day 2 _____ BPM

Day 3 _____ BPM

TOTAL FOR 3 DAYS: _____

POSTTEST

DATE _____

Day 1 _____ BPM

Day 2 _____ BPM

Day 3 _____ BPM

TOTAL FOR 3 DAYS: _____

Divide this total by 3 to determine your average resting heart rate.

PRETEST RESULTS

Average resting heart rate

_____ BPM

POSTTEST RESULTS

Average resting heart rate

_____ BPM

CALCULATING TARGET HEART RATE ZONE
USING THE MAXIMUM HEART RATE FORMULA

Name _____   Class Day/Time _____

Age _____

STEP 1
Calculate maximum heart rate (MHR) by subtracting your age from the number 226 if you are female or your age from the number 220 if you are male.

FEMALE   MALE
226 – age _____ = _____ MHR   220 – age _____ = _____ MHR

STEP 2
Determine your training heart rate zone by taking 60 percent (less fit) and 90 percent (very fit) of your MHR.

$$\underline{\hspace{3cm}} \times 60\% \text{ or } 0.6 = \underline{\hspace{3cm}}$$
MHR   low end of
                                           training zone

$$\underline{\hspace{3cm}} \times 90\% \text{ or } 0.9 = \underline{\hspace{3cm}}$$
MHR   high end of
                                           training zone

The range between these two percentages is where your heart rate should be while exercising. Depending upon your fitness level, you will want to work more toward one end or the other.

STEP 3
To determine your heart rate while exercising, use one of the following methods:

1. *6-second heart rate.* Take pulse for 6 seconds and multiply by 10.

$$\underline{\hspace{3cm}} \times 10 = \underline{\hspace{3cm}}$$
6-sec. pulse   heart rate

2. *10-second heart rate.* Take pulse for 10 seconds and multiply by 6.

$$\underline{\hspace{3cm}} \times 6 = \underline{\hspace{3cm}}$$
10-sec. pulse   heart rate

Whichever method you use, check that your heart rate, while you are exercising, remains within the training heart rate zone calculated in step 2.

CALCULATING YOUR TARGET HEART RATE ZONE USING KARVONEN'S FORMULA (FEMALE)   Name _____

Initial assessment date: _____
_____ resting heart rate

STEP I
Estimate your maximum heart rate by subtracting your age from 226.

226
− _____ age
_____ maximum heart rate

STEP II
Subtract your resting heart rate from your maximum heart rate.

_____ maximum heart rate
− _____ resting heart rate

STEP III
Multiply answer from Step II by

60% or 0.6 = _____
and by
90% or 0.9 = _____

STEP IV
To answers in Step III, add your resting heart rate.

_____ + _____ (resting heart rate) = _____
_____ + _____ (resting heart rate) = _____

The range between these two sums is your target training zone to use while exercising.

60% _____ to 90% _____

2nd assessment date: _____
_____ resting heart rate

STEP I
Estimate your maximum heart rate by subtracting your age from 226.

226
− _____ age
_____ maximum heart rate

STEP II
Subtract your resting heart rate from your maximum heart rate.

_____ maximum heart rate
− _____ resting heart rate

STEP III
Multiply answer from Step II by

60% or 0.6 = _____
and by
90% or 0.9 = _____

STEP IV
To answers in Step III, add your resting heart rate.

_____ + _____ (resting heart rate) = _____
_____ + _____ (resting heart rate) = _____

The range between these two sums is your target training zone to use while exercising.

60% _____ to 90% _____

End of semester date: _____
_____ resting heart rate

STEP I
Estimate your maximum heart rate by subtracting your age from 226.

226
− _____ age
_____ maximum heart rate

STEP II
Subtract your resting heart rate from your maximum heart rate.

_____ maximum heart rate
− _____ resting heart rate

STEP III
Multiply answer from Step II by

60% or 0.6 = _____
and by
90% or 0.9 = _____

STEP IV
To answers in Step III, add your resting heart rate.

_____ + _____ (resting heart rate) = _____
_____ + _____ (resting heart rate) = _____

The range between these two sums is your target training zone to use while exercising.

60% _____ to 90% _____

CALCULATING YOUR TARGET HEART RATE ZONE
USING KARVONEN'S FORMULA (MALE)   Name _____

Initial assessment date: _____	2nd assessment date: _____	End of semester date: _____
_____ resting heart rate	_____ resting heart rate	_____ resting heart rate

STEP I

Estimate your maximum heart rate by subtracting your age from 220.

220
− _____ age
_____ maximum heart rate

STEP II

Subtract your resting heart rate from your maximum heart rate.

_____ maximum heart rate
− _____ resting heart rate

STEP III

Multiply answer from Step II by

60% or 0.6 = _____
and by
90% or 0.9 = _____

STEP IV

To answers in Step III, add your resting heart rate.

_____ + _____ (resting heart rate) = _____
_____ + _____ (resting heart rate) = _____

The range between these two sums is your target training zone to use while exercising.

60% _____ to 90% _____

STEP I

Estimate your maximum heart rate by subtracting your age from 220.

220
− _____ age
_____ maximum heart rate

STEP II

Subtract your resting heart rate from your maximum heart rate.

_____ maximum heart rate
− _____ resting heart rate

STEP III

Multiply answer from Step II by

60% or 0.6 = _____
and by
90% or 0.9 = _____

STEP IV

To answers in Step III, add your resting heart rate.

_____ + _____ (resting heart rate) = _____
_____ + _____ (resting heart rate) = _____

The range between these two sums is your target training zone to use while exercising.

60% _____ to 90% _____

STEP I

Estimate your maximum heart rate by subtracting your age from 220.

220
− _____ age
_____ maximum heart rate

STEP II

Subtract your resting heart rate from your maximum heart rate.

_____ maximum heart rate
− _____ resting heart rate

STEP III

Multiply answer from Step II by

60% or 0.6 = _____
and by
90% or 0.9 = _____

STEP IV

To answers in Step III, add your resting heart rate.

_____ + _____ (resting heart rate) = _____
_____ + _____ (resting heart rate) = _____

The range between these two sums is your target training zone to use while exercising.

60% _____ to 90% _____

1.5-MILE RUN/3-MILE WALK TEST

1. Name _____ Sex _____ Age _____

2. Medical Clearance: No Restrictions _____ Restrictions _____

3. Physical Condition: Unconditioned beginner _____

                   Conditioned beginner _____

4. **PHYSICAL CONDITION**   **TEST CLEARANCE**   **SUGGESTION**

    No medical clearance   No   Get medical examination.

    Unconditioned beginner   No   Complete beginner's program.

    Conditioned beginner   Yes

    Test Clearance: Yes _____   No _____

    If no: Subject must have a medical exam. _____

    Subject must complete beginner's program. _____

5. Test: 1.5-mile run _____ 3-mile walk _____

6. When test will be held _____ Where _____

7. Time for 1.5-mile run _____ Time for 3-mile walk _____

8. Fitness Category: _____ I. Very Poor _____ III. Fair   _____ V. Excellent

                     _____ II. Poor   _____ IV. Good   _____ VI. Superior

(Table of fitness categories on the following page.)

FITNESS CATEGORIES FOR THE 1.5-MILE RUN/3-MILE WALK TEST

(These tables give times in minutes and seconds.)

1.5-MILE RUN TEST
Age (years)

Fitness Category		13–19	20–29	30–39	40–49	50–59	60+
I. Very Poor	(men)	>15:31	>16:01	>16:31	>17:31	>19:01	20:01
	(women)	>18:31	>19:01	>19:31	>20:01	>20:31	21:01
II. Poor	(men)	12:11-15:30	14:01-16:00	14:44-16:30	15:36-17:30	17:01-19:00	19:01-20:00
	(women)	16:55-18:30	18:31-19:00	19:01-19:30	19:31-20:00	20:01-20:30	20:31-21:00
III. Fair	(men)	10:49-12:10	12:01-14:00	12:31-14:45	13:01-15:35	14:31-17:00	16:16-19:00
	(women)	14:31-16:54	15:55-18:30	16:31-19:00	17:31-19:30	19:01-20:00	19:31-20:30
IV. Good	(men)	9:41-10:48	10:46-12:00	11:01-12:30	11:31-13:00	12:31-14:30	14:00-16:15
	(women)	12:30-14:30	13:31-15:54	14:31-16:30	15:56-17:30	16:31-19:00	17:31-19:30
V. Excellent	(men)	8:37-9:40	9:45-10:45	10:00-11:00	10:30-11:30	11:00-12:30	11:15-13:59
	(women)	11:50-12:29	12:30-13:30	13:00-14:30	13:45-15:55	14:30-16:30	16:30-17:30
VI. Superior	(men)	<8:37	<9:45	<10:00	<10:30	<11:00	<11:15
	(women)	<11:50	<12:30	<13:00	<13:45	<14:30	<16:30

3-MILE WALKING TEST (NO RUNNING)
Age (years)

Fitness Category		13–19	20–29	30–39	40–49	50–59	60+
I. Very Poor	(men)	>45:00	>46:00	>49:00	>52:00	>55:00	>60:00
	(women)	>47:00	>48:00	>51:00	>54:00	>57:00	>63:00
II. Poor	(men)	41:01-45:00	42:01-46:00	44:31-49:00	47:01-52:00	50:01-55:00	54:01-60:00
	(women)	43:01-47:00	44:01-48:00	46:31-51:00	49:01-54:00	52:01-57:00	57:01-63:00
III. Fair	(men)	37:31-41:00	38:31-42:00	40:01-44:30	42:01-47:00	45:01-50:00	48:01-54:00
	(women)	39:31-43:00	40:31-44:00	42:01-46:30	44:01-49:00	47:01-52:00	51:01-57:00
IV. Good	(men)	33:00-37:30	34:00-38:30	35:00-40:00	36:30-42:00	39:00-45:00	41:00-48:00
	(women)	35:00-39:30	36:00-40:30	37:30-42:00	39:00-44:00	42:00-47:00	45:00-51:00
V. Excellent	(men)	<33:00	<34:00	<35:00	<36:30	<39:00	<41:00
	(women)	<35:00	<36:00	<37:30	<39:00	<42:00	<45:00

3-MINUTE STEP TEST

The step test is used to measure the recovery heart rate as a means of evaluating an individual's cardiorespiratory fitness level. Stepping on and off a bench for 3 minutes at a selected cadence will give an estimate of a person's capacity for hard work. The faster that the heart recovers from the bout of standardized exercise, the higher the fitness rating. Though a laboratory-administered maximal oxygen uptake test is more accurate for testing cardiorespiratory endurance, the step test is much more feasible. It can be given to individuals or large groups. It serves not only as a screening test but also as a standard by which training progress can be monitored. This simple test should be administered in pairs: a timer and a stepper. Minimal equipment is required: a locker-room bench or bleacher, a watch, and a card for record keeping. Also useful is a metronome or cadence tape.

PROCEDURE

1. Participants should be well rested and not have engaged in aerobic exercise the day of the test. The height of the bench should be between 12–18 inches, and the stepping cadence from 96 to 120 steps per minute. These variations do not appear to affect the test results.

2. Participants step up with the left foot, up with right foot, then down with left foot and down with right foot. It is suggested that the lead leg change during the test. The cadence is most easily kept with a metronome or a prepared audio tape. The four-count phrase (up up down down) should take $2–2^1/_2$ seconds to complete, for a total of 24 to 30 sets in 1 minute. Continue stepping for 3 minutes.

3. After 3 minutes the participant sits down and the timer takes the stepper's pulse for 1 *full minute*. Remember, it is the recovery rate and not the exercise heart rate that is being measured.

General recovery heart rate ratings are as follows (BPM = beats per minute):

Superior to excellent	<90 BPM
Good to average	90–100 BPM
Fair	101–120 BPM
Poor	>120 BPM

National Dance-Exercise Instructor Training Association (NDEITA), 1505 South Washington Ave., Suite 208, Minneapolis, MN 55454. Reebok International, Ltd. *Introduction to Step Reebok*, 1991.

ABDOMINAL TESTS

To assess the endurance of the abdominal muscles, perform the sit-up test or the curl-up test.

THE 60-SECOND SIT-UP TEST

Do not take this test if you suffer from low-back pain.

EQUIPMENT

1. Stopwatch, clock, or watch with a second hand

2. Partner to hold your ankles

3. Mat or towel to lie on (optional)

PREPARATION
Try a few sit-ups to get used to the proper technique and warm up your abdominal muscles.

INSTRUCTIONS

1. Lie flat on your back on the floor with knees bent, feet flat on the floor, and your fingers interlocked behind your neck. Your partner should hold your ankles firmly so that your feet stay on the floor as you do the sit-ups.

2. When someone signals you to begin, raise your head and chest off the floor until your elbows touch your knees or thighs, and then return to the starting position. Keep your neck neutral. Keep your breathing as normal as possible; don't hold your breath.

3. Perform as many sit-ups as you can in 60 seconds.

Note: The norms for this test were established with subjects interlocking their fingers behind their neck; your results will be most accurate if you use this technique. However, some experts feel that sit-ups done in this position can cause injury to the neck. If this is a concern, perform the test with your hands cupped over your ears rather than behind your neck. Alternatively, complete the curl-up test described later in this lab. If you perform sit-ups with your hands behind your neck, take care not to force your neck forward, and stop if you feel any pain in your neck.

Number of sit-ups: _____

(continued on next page)

ABDOMINAL TESTS (CONTINUED)

RATING YOUR MUSCULAR ENDURANCE
Refer to the table below for a rating of your abdominal muscle endurance. Record
your rating below and in the fitness profile.

Rating:_____

RATINGS FOR THE 60-SECOND SIT-UP TEST

NUMBER OF SIT-UPS

MEN	VERY POOR	POOR	FAIR	GOOD	EXCELLENT	SUPERIOR
Age: Under 20	Below 36	36–40	41–46	47–50	51–61	Above 61
20–29	Below 33	33–37	38–41	42–46	47–54	Above 54
30–39	Below 30	30–34	35–38	39–42	43–50	Above 50
40–49	Below 24	24–28	29–33	34–38	39–46	Above 46
50–59	Below 19	19–23	24–27	28–34	35–42	Above 42
60 and over	Below 15	15–18	19–21	22–29	30–38	Above 38
WOMEN	**VERY POOR**	**POOR**	**FAIR**	**GOOD**	**EXCELLENT**	**SUPERIOR**
Age: Under 20	Below 28	28–31	32–35	36–45	46–54	Above 54
20–29	Below 24	24–31	32–37	38–43	44–50	Above 50
30–39	Below 20	20–24	25–28	29–34	35–41	Above 41
40–49	Below 14	14–19	20–23	24–28	29–37	Above 37
50–59	Below 10	10–13	14–19	20–23	24–29	Above 29
60 and over	Below 3	3–5	6–10	11–16	17–27	Above 27

Source: Based on norms from the Cooper Institute for Aerobics Research, Dallas, Texas; used with permission.

(continued on next page)

ABDOMINAL TESTS (CONTINUED)

THE CURL-UP TEST

The rationale for using curl-ups in place of sit-ups is convincing. In a full sit-up, part of the lift is provided by the hip-flexors muscles. Curl-ups optimize the use of the abdominal muscles, and for that reason curl-ups are routinely used in fitness classes.

EQUIPMENT

1. Metronome

2. Stopwatch, clock, or watch with a second hand

3. Heavy tape

4. Ruler

5. Partner

6. Mat (optional)

PREPARATION

1. Set the metronome at a rate of 50 beats per minute.

2. Place a tape strip approximately 1 meter long on the floor or mat. Place another strip of tape 10 centimeters away from the first one.

INSTRUCTIONS

1. Start by laying on your back on the floor, arms by your sides, palms down and on the floor, elbows locked, and fingers straight. The longest fingertip of each hand should touch the edge of the near strip of tape. Your knees should be bent at about 90 degrees, with your feet 12–18 inches away from your buttocks.

2. To perform a curl-up, curl your head and upper back upward, keeping your arms straight. Slide your fingertips forward along the floor until you touch the other strip of tape, 10 centimeters from the starting position. Then curl back down so that your upper back and head touch the floor. Palms, feet, and buttocks should stay on the floor throughout the curl-up. (For this test, your partner does not hold your feet.) Maintain the 90-degree angle in your knees. Exhale during the lift phase of the curl-up.

3. Start the metronome at the correct cadence. You will perform curl-ups at the steady, continuous rate of 25 per minute. Curl up on one beat and curl down on the next. Your partner counts the number of curl-ups you complete and makes sure that you maintain correct form.

(continued on next page)

ABDOMINAL TESTS (CONTINUED)

4. Perform as many curl-ups as you can in one minute. If at any point during the test you can no longer maintain proper form and keep up with the rhythm set by the metronome, stop the test and record the number of curl-ups you performed up to that point.

Number of curl-ups: _____

RATING YOUR MUSCULAR ENDURANCE
Your score is the number of completed curl-ups. Refer to the appropriate portion of the table below for a rating of your abdominal muscular endurance. Record your rating below and in the fitness profile.

Rating:_____

RATINGS FOR THE CURL-UP TEST

NUMBER OF CURL-UPS

MEN	Needs Improvement	Fair	Good	Very Good	Excellent
Age: 15–19	Below 16	16–20	21–22	23–24	25
20–29	Below 13	13–20	21–22	23–24	25
30–39	Below 13	13–20	21–22	23–24	25
40–49	Below 11	11–15	16–21	22–24	25
50–59	Below 9	9–13	14–19	20–24	25
60–69	Below 4	4–9	10–15	16–24	25
WOMEN	Needs Improvement	Fair	Good	Very Good	Excellent
Age: 15–19	Below 16	16–20	21–22	23–24	25
20–29	Below 13	13–18	19–22	23–24	25
30–39	Below 11	11–15	16–21	22–24	25
40–49	Below 6	6–12	13–20	21–24	25
50–59	Below 4	4–8	9–15	16–24	25
60–69	Below 2	2–5	6–10	11–17	18–25

Source: *The Canadian Physical Activity, Fitness and Lifestyle Appraisal: CSEP's Plan for Healthy Active Living*, 1996. Reprinted by permission of the Canadian Society for Exercise Physiology.

PUSH-UP TEST

EQUIPMENT

1. Partner

2. Mat or towel (for knees during modified push-ups)

3. Pencil or pen

DIRECTIONS

1. Warm up and stretch, especially arms and chest.

2. Decide whether you will be performing regular or modified push-ups. (Regular push-ups are performed on hands and toes, modified push-ups are performed on hands and knees.) The norms for modified push-ups are based on a female population, whereas the norms for regular push-ups are based on a male population. (Either gender may perform either test as long as it is understood that so far no norms have been compiled for females doing regular push-ups and males performing modified push-ups.)

3. To begin this test, lie on your stomach, legs together. Position your hands under your shoulders with fingers pointing forward. On the start signal push up from the mat, fully extending your elbows, and then lower down until your chin touches the mat. Your chest and abdomen should not touch the floor. You must maintain a straight body alignment at all times. Your partner will count only correctly completed push-ups.

4. There is no time limit on this test. Perform as many correct push-ups as you can without taking a break. The test will be stopped when you strain forcibly or are unable to maintain correct technique over two repetitions.

5. Record the number of correct push-ups you complete.
   _____ push-ups   Circle one: Regular   Modified

6. Consult the norms below and record your fitness level. (Fill in an "X" if there are no gender-appropriate norms for the test position you selected.)
   _____ fitness rating

7. Stretch your arms and chest muscles to prevent soreness.

Norms by age groups and gender for push-ups.*

	AGE (YEARS)											
FITNESS	**15–19**		**20–29**		**30–39**		**40–49**		**50–59**		**60–69**	
RATING	**M**	**F**	**M**	**F**	**M**	**F**	**M**	**F**	**M**	**F**	**M**	**F**
Excellent	≥39	≥33	≥36	≥30	≥30	≥27	≥22	≥24	≥21	≥21	≥18	≥17
Above Average	29–38	25–32	29–35	21–29	22–29	20–26	17–21	15–23	13–20	11–20	11–17	12–16
Average	23–28	18–24	22–28	15–20	17–21	13–19	13–16	11–14	10–12	7–10	8–10	5–11
Below Average	18–22	12–17	17–21	10–14	12–16	8–12	10–12	5–10	7–9	2–6	5–7	1–4
Poor	≤17	≤11	≤16	≤9	≤11	≤7	≤9	≤4	≤6	≤1	≤4	≤1

* Based on data from the Canada Fitness Survey. 1981.

From: *The Canadian Standardized Test of Fitness Manual*, 3rd Edition 1986. Used with permission from the Canadian Society for Exercise Physiology in cooperation with Fitness Canada–Health Canada.

SELF-TEST FLEXIBILITY EVALUATIONS

In an overall fitness assessment procedure the participant would, of course, have both upper and lower body flexibility evaluated. Because this text pertains to bench stepping, the flexibility tests discussed here will be to assess the participant's range of motion in those areas that directly affect their ability to engage in bench stepping for aerobic exercise. Prior to beginning a bench stepping program, it is important to evaluate the range of motion to the lower back, quadriceps, hamstrings, and calf area.

Before beginning each test it is important to relax the muscle. Also, participants should be told not to bounce into a position or force their body beyond reasonable limits. There should be no pain. Participants should note whether they are able to achieve a "passing" position.

QUADRICEPS

Participant lies prone with knees together and gently brings one heel to the buttocks.

Passing: The heel should touch the buttocks.

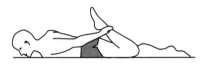

CALVES (GASTRONCNEMIUS/SOLEUS)

Participant stands with toes on a thick block or book (2 inches) and slowly lowers heels toward the floor.

Passing: The heels should touch the floor.

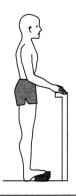

LOWER BACK

Participant lies on back and pulls both knees up to the chest.

Passing: Both knees should touch the chest.

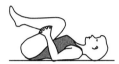

HIP FLEXOR (ILIOPSOAS)

Participant lies on back with one knee pulled to the chest, the other leg fully extended to the floor.

Passing: The calf of the extended leg must remain on the floor with the knee straight.

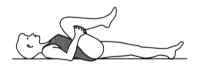

HAMSTRINGS

Participant lies on back and lifts one leg while keeping the other leg fully extended on the floor. The knee of the leg on the floor must be straight.

Passing: The raised leg should reach vertical position.

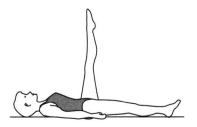

PERSONAL FITNESS LOG

Name ——————————————————— Day ——— Time ——— Class ———

Keep this log for activities outside aerobics class.

DATE	ACTIVITY	DISTANCE	TIME/DURATION	PULSE RATE

Instructor remarks:

NAME _____ Section _____ Date _____

NUTRITION LOG

Keep a record of everything you eat for three consecutive days. Record all food and beverage intake. Evaluate the food item in its simplest form. For example, a roast beef sandwich would be recorded as 2 slices of bread, 3 oz. of roast beef, and 1 Tbsp. of mayonnaise. At the end of the day, use the Food Guide Pyramid (Table 7-2) to analyze your daily diet.

FOOD	NUMBER OF SERVINGS	FOOD GROUP

FOOD PYRAMID ANALYSIS

FOOD GROUP	NUMBER OF SERVINGS
Milk, yogurt, cheese	
Meat, poultry, fish, dry beans, eggs, nuts	
Fruits	
Vegetables	
Bread, cereals, rice, pasta	

INDEX